I'm Not Drunk ...
I Just Have MS

*my incredible journey with, and
recovery from, multiple sclerosis*

Bruce Pelham

ISBN   978-0-9851725-0-3

For ordering information, please visit:

www.myMScure.com

or

order by mail at:

P. O. Box 14301

Tallahassee, FL 32308

Add $4.00 S&H

<u>Dedication</u>

To Kathy Raynor, my friend and teacher.

From the three years I served with you as a sponsor for our young people through your most recent health challenge, I have been blessed.

To know you; to have you as a friend; to learn from you.

Godspeed on your journey as you continue to create miracles.

Acknowledgments

To my typist and editor, Marti Hildebrandt, and my editor, Boyd L. Merritt, without whom this book may never have been completed, I extend my gratitude and appreciation.

ITINERARY
(Introduction)

> *The act of writing is the act of discovering what you believe.*   *-- David Hare*

Sometimes a book is written to record events as they happened, from the author's point-of-view. Sometimes it is written to pass along that information to others. Some people theorize that it is always written for the benefit of the author. It has been referred to as the act of discovering what you believe.

My purpose in writing this book included all of these. From the beginning of my journey with multiple sclerosis I made notes about what was going on with me, both mentally and physically. To begin with, it was to make sure I could remember the details for my next visit with my doctor. Then it was for me to track my progress. Little did I know at the time, what a challenging journey it would be.

For the past several years, I intended to write this book. I spent increasingly more time making notes to myself as I recalled various aspects of my experience. My neurologist, Dr. Charles G. Maitland, observed me through this entire process, from the beginning. He was nothing short of wonderful. He was honest and direct about what was happening with me. He endured my reluctance to take medicine for multiple sclerosis and continued as my doctor anyway. I will discuss that more fully later in the book.

When I became really serious about writing the book, I asked him for my records, starting from the beginning of my treatment. At the end of each visit, he would dictate a summary of his observations. His staff copied that summary of each visit beginning with my first visit in December of 1992. Actually, they did that twice because I misplaced the first set of copies. I mention this because it is indicative of the problems I had with one of my most troublesome symptoms, the sporadic loss of short term recall. For purposes of my story, it was important to me that it be as factually accurate as I could make it. I knew I could not correctly recall all of the events, as to the facts or the dates.

> *Although the world is full of suffering, it is also full of the overcoming of it.*
>
> *-- Helen Keller*

It is a story of much mental and physical suffering; fortunately only a few moments of great despair; and a journey of physical and mental rehabilitation. It was a journey of faith and determination. It was about recognizing that ultimately I could affect many of the things going on with my body. Just as an athlete could fine tune his (or her) body to perform at a high level, so could I. It is just that my starting point was a bit different.

At my lowest ebb, I was a physical and mental wreck. I was unemployable for three years and almost totally dependent on friends and family. My body was a total wreck from the disease that made a home in my body. My immune system was, to say the least, deficient. Today, few people would notice that I have, or had, multiple sclerosis.

> *The journey is your goal and your work is your path.*   *-- Lao Tzu*

This book is about my journey with multiple sclerosis and of my thoughts about causes and treatment. Answers, for the most part, are theories and nothing more. I have borrowed heavily from existing medical research. I came across a quote from an unknown source that I found to be appropriate. "To steal ideas from one person is plagiarism. To steal from many is research."

Giving individual credit to the many researchers and writers on this subject would simply have made my task more cumbersome and the book less readable. I greatly appreciate all of the work that has been done and opinions offered, in looking for cures and explanations. I don't pretend to be one of those people. My book is about my own experience. All of the information about the disease is offered so that my story will be meaningful.

My purpose is that it provide hope for those diagnosed with multiple sclerosis and for the people involved in their lives. Many of the principles discussed in this book are equally applicable to other illnesses. I encourage readers, and potential readers, to look at the book with this in mind.

Much of my research was done before I seriously contemplated writing this book. It was done to help me understand what was happening to me. With much of the material, I wouldn't even have known the source except that, in a general sense, it came from the internet, books, and articles.

A great deal of what I knew about "searching the web" was learned by trial and error as I looked for information on what was going on with me. There is simply no way to express the gratitude I feel toward all of those people from whom I have borrowed; the researchers who have looked for a cause and treatment; the doctors who have attempted to provide some relief from this unpredictable disease; and the MS patients and their families who have shared what goes on with them and whose lives have been touched in a very real way.

> *We are divine enough to ask and are important enough to receive.*
> *-- Dr. Wayne Dyer*

I invite you to consider the things that you alone can do to affect the path the disease takes with your mind and body. I look at how it affected mine; starting with the horrific debilitation of my mind and body, to the point where my symptoms have disappeared or, are hardly noticeable. I asked God to take the disease from me and to guide me in knowing what to do to make this happen. I began my miles of walking, accompanied by the slow but steady progress I made in rebuilding my body and rewiring my mind. Never believe for one

> *When the solution is simple, God is answering.* -- *Albert Einstein*

minute that there is no hope. That, along with your attitude, can accomplish great things. Asking God's help seems too simple sometimes.

The things accomplished because some great mind conceived them are too numerous to list. Think of the Wright brothers as they pictured a plane flying through the air, before a plane ever existed. Think of Edison as he had several hundred "failures" on the way to inventing the light bulb. Think of Einstein pondering the Theory of Relativity before anyone had ever considered its existence. To succeed, you must be willing to fail; to fall flat on your face, literally and figuratively. I am reminded of Babe Ruth who was quick to point out that his home runs came because he was willing to strike out. Dr. Bernie Siegel, M.D., a prominent physician and now a writer, voiced a similar thought when he asked whether one would rather step up to the plate and take a swing or watch from the sideline.

Dr. Siegel tells of a cancer patient who was terminally ill. After being told he had only a few months left to live, that patient stopped coming to see him. Dr. Siegel ran into him on the street many years later after having thought all of this time that the man was deceased.

He asked the man to come to his office for an examination and found no signs of cancer. He was amazed, of course, and asked the man what had happened.

The man said, very simply, "You told me I was dying and didn't have long to live. I wasn't ready to die and so I saw no reason to come back and listen to any more of that. I had too many things left to do, and here I am, still doing them."

Stories like these are discounted by lots of people. And that includes a lot of educated people. All too often, they are the biggest skeptics of all. They are too intelligent to believe such stories, always thinking there must be some logical explanation that we just do not see. Our body is capable of so much more than our conscious mind imagines. There are many examples of "miracles" – things we cannot explain.

My neurologist, forever a bright star to me in the field of medicine, openly admits to having no medical explanation for my recovery. In all of his years of practice, he has never had a case that parallels mine, nor has he known of one. This is a doctor with many years in the field, a practitioner who serves on the faculty at the Florida State University School of Medicine.

If you believe that you can affect the outcome, you can. ***THIS IS THE MOST IMPORTANT MESSAGE IN THIS BOOK.*** The alternative is for you to believe that there is nothing you can do except to take medicine and wait. This alternative is a route that may ensure its own destination. It is all about attitude and what you believe.

> *Life is an attitude. It's what you believe, always.*   *-- Dr. Wayne Dyer*

People have different symptoms and respond differently to different medicines and treatments. It is so easy to say, "But mine is different," because it is. It is easy for you to prove me wrong. And THEN, you get to be right.

When my two daughters were both expecting sons, I made a decision to live closer to them at some point while the boys were growing up. My grandparents were an important part of my life. Grandparents add something special, including when there are good parents. I wanted to be around to add that "something."

I practiced administrative law for the State of Florida for many years. I couldn't envision doing that in a different state. I decided to go back to school instead. The University of Florida has one of the top law schools, nationally, for providing an L.L.M. degree in taxation. It is widely considered to be one of the top two such schools in the country.

You can't go around being what everyone expects you to be, living your life through other people's rules, and be happy and have inner peace. *--Dr. Wayne Dyer*

I knew if I got that degree, I could go to Atlanta, or anywhere else, and practice tax law. Not the most exciting thing I could imagine, but one that would greatly improve my prospects in a new city and state, and allow me to be closer to my grandkids.

When I started this process, of course, I had the normal doubts and fears one might expect from a 63 year old applying to be a student at what is considered to be one of the top programs of its kind in the entire country. Admittedly, it felt great to be accepted. I knew it would be difficult. I can't remember any subject that I had in law school being more difficult than taxation, and that was forty years ago. Auditing classes at Florida State University College of Law for a semester, in preparation for doing this, reminded me of just how difficult it would be.

Never one to shy away from a challenge, I was convinced that I could do it. I was auditing 10 hours which quickly became a full-time job. I was still working half-time, which I tried for a while. Eventually, I gave up working completely to devote full-time to studying. This was before I even knew I was accepted at the University of

Florida. I was determined to make this happen and "knew" that I could. My co-workers honored me with a "going away" breakfast, and the following day I received my acceptance from the University of Florida.

Going to Gainesville to look for a place to live was exhilarating. I was excited at being around students and at the prospect of doing something different and challenging. It was invigorating.

Nothing is more powerful than an idea whose time has come. -- Victor Hugo

On the way back from that first trip to Gainesville I felt a tug inside. It turned into a full-fledged struggle during the following week. It wasn't the fear of giving up the security of my job. I had already calculated that I could survive while I was going to school, have health insurance as a retiree until I reached Medicare age, and would start drawing Social Security eventually. After school, I was planning to teach and practice. I planned to work and be productive long past what would be considered a normal retirement age. The struggle going on inside was about something else.

For a long time I have intended to write this book about my journey with multiple sclerosis. Everyone has some kind of story. Some good and some not so good. Most never get written. In the words of Oliver Wendell Holmes, "Many of us die with music still inside."

Only a life lived for others is a life worthwhile.   *-- Albert Einstein*

I think my story will benefit many people, especially those with the disease and those close to someone with the disease. For years, I have made notes of my own experiences. I have collected files from all my years of visits with my neurologist and had lots of thoughts about this project rolling around in my head. It is just that working full-time and taking care of everyday living had not left time to write. There was a forty hour work week; going to and from work; exercising and walking most days; doing routine, everyday kinds of errands and essentials (cleaners, laundry, car maintenance, eating); visiting my daughters, Lori and Shelley, and their families once in a while; getting to visit and watch FSU sports with Mom; and an occasional outing with friends. I was reminded frequently that it takes courage to make decisions with which others disagree.

> *We need to have the courage and openness*
> *to revise a plan if a new one seems better.*
> *-- Alan Cohen*

The struggle that raged inside me for days was simply, "Do I spend the next eighteen months studying tax, not the most exciting, inspiring course of study in the universe, or, do I write the book I have intended, for so long, to write?" After days of agony and silent meditation, the clarity finally came in the form of a question. "If I were on my death bed, would I be wishing that I could have studied tax for the last eighteen months?" The answer was, very clearly, NO.

Or, in the alternative, would I be thinking, "I wish I had taken the time to write my book." The answer was, very clearly, YES. The struggle going on inside instantly subsided and, for the first time, I felt peace. No longer was I struggling with regret at not having written this book.

Regret for the things we did can be tempered by time; it is regret for the things we did not do that is inconsolable.
-- Sydney J. Harris

My return trip to Gainesville that week was for a meeting with the head of the L.L.M. program, Professor Friel, for orientation. I had to explain why I wasn't going to be there in the fall. I could have written or I could have called. I was so grateful for having had the opportunity to study there, however, that it was important to explain why I would not be coming and that I do that in person.

Let him that would move the world, first move himself. *--Socrates*

We talked for a long time. He could not have been more gracious, more understanding, or more supportive. He understood my need to write the book and my need to come talk to him. After I had told him about my decision-making process, he told me another similar story.

Years ago, he was watching a special on Public Television about the same kind of decision. What he had always remembered from that story was that "few, if any, people on their death beds are wishing they had gotten back to the office to finish that project they were working on."

He said, "I have just one, important favor to ask of you." He handed me his card and said, "When you get your book published, will you call me and tell me where I can buy a copy?" I knew I had been in the presence of a really special person. He understood that I was making the right decision for me and doing what I needed to do.

> *All of us are on our own paths, doing*
> *exactly what we know how to do at the*
> *moment, given the conditions of our lives.*
> *-- Dr. Wayne Dyer*

Chapter 1

Off We Go
(Beginning Symptoms)

Symptoms, then, are in reality, nothing but the cry from suffering organs.
-- Jean-Martin Charcot

I was working with a state agency when I first noticed unusual things going on with my body. Our office was located in a typical multi-story office building in the downtown area.

For days on end I worked long hours. I would work until everybody went home, get some dinner, and work some more. A part of this was due to my longstanding workaholic work habits. My dad had been a hard worker, to the extreme, and had passed this workaholism on to me and to each of my siblings. And part of it was due to my observations that so many people, particularly my superiors, were overworked. I thought that if I did more, my supervisor would not have quite so much to do.

It didn't surprise me that my supervisor noticed how much work I was producing. It did surprise me that he had some idea about the long hours I was working. Many times when I came in on the weekends, he would be there working. He had been there many years and, of course, he had some idea about how long certain jobs should take. He made the assignments and had ready access to my assignment sheet. He could easily see when I was opening and closing files.

Still, it surprised me when he finally said something. We were waiting for the elevator at the same time one day and nobody else was around. I have always remembered him saying, "Bruce, I really do appreciate all of the work that you do. And I appreciate why you do it. But one thing you really do need to understand. The more work we turn out, the more they give me to get done. I never get caught up."

When he said that, it was as if he was reading my mind and always knew what I was doing. He was a great supervisor. He was firm when he needed to be, expected his attorneys to make decisions, and was always supportive. His people were important to him.

My work habits were made possible by an incredibly talented and loyal legal assistant. She had been there over thirty years. She was incredibly competent, a pleasure to work with, and helped me to manage a heavy caseload that kept us both busy. She knew more about my job than I did.

In my early years with the department, I never took a single case to hearing. There wasn't time. Taking a case to hearing would take several days; collecting exhibits, preparing the case for hearing, writing proposed orders and all the while my cases would be piling up.

I was a good negotiator from all my years in business. I had to make sure the attorneys for the insurance companies "knew" without me saying that I was ready to go to hearing at the "drop of a hat." With me knowing, of course, that

I simply did not have time to take a case to hearing. Some of the cases were about little more than routine matters. Others were complicated, involving lots of money and violations of the law. These sometimes took weeks to resolve.

Eventually, my supervisor was asked to head another department, out of the Legal section. The attorney who replaced him as my supervisor was a good friend as well as co-worker before his promotion. For a while I continued to perform well. Then things began to change.

I do not remember how long I had been aware of the unusual things going on with me before discussing them with anyone. In retrospect, I am quite sure that I had been aware of them for at least a year as they progressed and probably more. I knew that my work habits had kept me from facing the seriousness of what was going on with me. I should have realized, of course, that "symptoms" are usually cries for help from an ailing body.

The most noticeable initial symptom came when I would be performing the simple task, normally, of walking down the hallway. As I walked I veered toward the left wall. I would, unconsciously for the most part, reach out and touch the wall on my left side. This was to keep me from running into the wall.

Eventually, I would be pushing off from the wall with every step that I took. By then, it was very noticeable to me. I "knew" something was wrong and wasn't so sure that I wanted to know what. Many of us, and men in particular, let egos get in the way. We avoid finding out for fear that something really is wrong. I was no exception.

Sure, I wondered what was causing it. I made excuses to myself such as, I was really tired. Many times that was true. Then there were many times it happened when I was not tired.

Shortly before I started feeling really fatigued, in the summer of 1992, I taught a course in the evening at the local community college. This just added to an already heavy workload. I did it because it seemed like a fun way to subsidize the low salary made by attorneys for the state.

I only taught for one quarter. My fatigue, by then, was becoming really problematic. I taught two nights each week. That meant two more nights of preparation for class. I would be really dragging by the end of the class. It never occurred to me that this feeling of exhaustion was caused by something seriously wrong with me. But, I did not attempt teaching another course.

These things, I eventually learned, were symptoms of multiple sclerosis. When I looked back at the seriousness of some of these symptoms, I was amazed at how long it had taken me to go see a doctor to find out what was causing them. The symptoms are there to get our attention. They finally got mine.

As time passed, the fatigue was more and more noticeable. I worked so much that it didn't surprise me when I was tired. It helped to mask what was really going on with my body. Symptoms of what I later learned was multiple sclerosis, were becoming more noticeable and more troubling.

I was at work one morning in late 1992, and felt really weak, a sick feeling. I left to go home. About two miles from the office, I came to a park with a small lake. I was feeling so bad that I pulled in and parked. It was over 90 degrees at the time, but I had not yet realized how detrimental heat was to me.

I got out of my car and lay on the ground in the shade of a large oak. The heat totally finished me. I was still lying there eight hours later, as it was getting dark. I had slept intermittently, but had been awake most of the time and very uncomfortable in that heat. I was amazed when I thought about it later. This was a public park and no one had even checked to see if I was okay. Finally, it had cooled enough for me to have the energy to get up and go home. Heat exhaustion was one of many things I could not avoid noticing.

I began having more difficulty speaking. I couldn't quite say certain words. Initially, it would just be a word here and there. Then, my tongue would sometimes feel a little thick. One day I was talking on the phone with an attorney from out of town. We had been friends since the early grade school years. After high school, we were classmates in the major portion of undergraduate school and in law school. After law school, he did a four-year stint in the Air Force, but we always stayed in touch, so he knew me well.

That day on the phone, he asked, "How much have you had to drink?" I responded, "Nothing in years, why?" "Because you sound like you are drunk," he said. I remember realizing that what I had been hearing in my voice was obvious to everyone else as well. It wasn't something that I was hiding from anyone, especially from me.

Not only was my speech becoming slurred, but my balance was off and I felt very unstable at times. Heat was a major problem for me. The hotter it was, the more fatigued I became. My thinking process was slowing. I knew something wasn't as it should be.

The clincher came one day when I was going to use the phone. My memory of phone numbers was better than that of anyone I ever knew. I don't know how many phone numbers I had stored in my head, but dozens at least.

It was different from a photographic memory. Mine was based on understanding. I had noticed it when taking math courses in high school. It would often take a lot of hard work to understand something but once I did, it was "there." That is the way it was with phone numbers for me.

If I had called you once, even years before, I probably had your number safely "stashed away upstairs" with a picture of you. I rarely had to use a phone book. If I thought of calling you and picked up the phone, the number was there. I would usually dial it without even thinking about it.

That particular day, I reached for the phone, thinking of the person I was about to call and … no phone number. I placed the phone gently back in the cradle. I sat there for a minute puzzling over what had just happened. I could not even remember when anything like that had ever occurred. I decided I must have really been preoccupied with something.

Finally, I tried it again. The result was the same. I held the phone to my ear and my fingers prepared to dial … nothing. My mind was blank. My fingers didn't move. This time, I knew that something was terribly wrong.

That day in late 1992, I called a friend and asked him if he had noticed anything strange about me recently. He said, "Wait right there," and came over to my house immediately to talk with me.

He said his wife had remarked to him a few weeks prior that I sounded like I had been drinking. She knew that I had given that up many years before or she would have thought that I was. We discussed other things that he had noticed, like my walking difficulties and the movement of my eyes not "tracking." He had me promise that I would call my doctor first thing the next morning and get an appointment to go in and explain what had been happening. The next day I called for an appointment.

Chapter 2

Looking for a Road Map
(Search for an Answer)

We have forgotten the age-old fact that God speaks chiefly through dreams and visions. -- C. G. Jung

I never forgot that appointment with Dr. Van Sickle. I had only seen him once before, and that is when I had been assigned to him by my HMO.

Dr. Van Sickle was tremendous. When I went to see him, I had long since been amazed by how little time doctors spend with their patients. I asked him to just sit and listen as I told him what had been going on with me. I was reminded of that meeting years later when he said, "The patient always knows more about what's wrong than the doctor does. My job is to listen and see if I can figure out what that is so I can help."

He sat and listened. It seemed like 30 or 45 minutes that I talked, explaining all of the strange things that had been happening to me physically and mentally. He asked very few questions during all of that time. When I finally finished, he said that he could not tell me what the problem was. He wanted me to see a neurologist right away.

His office set up an appointment with Dr. Maitland and I saw him very quickly. He was just as attentive as Dr. Van Sickle had been. He started a series of tests which he gave me over the next few months. After that first visit, I saw him eight more times during the following year.

There wasn't then, and isn't now, a blood test for multiple sclerosis. This would simplify things, of course, and scientists have long worked on such a test. Analysis of blood is used to eliminate certain things. The imperfect system we have for its diagnosis involves eliminating other possibilities. A neurologist is normally the person to do that.

Approximately ten percent of patients diagnosed with multiple sclerosis have some other condition instead. Those diseases have some of the same symptoms which causes some of the difficulty in diagnosing. These conditions include inflammation of the blood vessels, multiple strokes, vitamin deficiency, brain infection, and lupus. Various tests and procedures are helpful in eliminating possibilities, and none are conclusive. These include MRIs, lumbar punctures or spinal taps, and different evoked potentials tests which help determine whether MS has affected a person's nerves.

In September 1993, Dr. Maitland recommended a lumbar puncture, or spinal tap, to confirm his suspected diagnosis that I had a demyelinating disease. He also recommended starting Beta Interferon. We waited on both.

The generally accepted criteria for diagnosing multiple sclerosis rely to a great extent on the ability and knowledge of the neurologist. MS usually begins in patients between 20-50 years of age. Certain symptoms indicate disease of the brain or spinal cord. Two or more lesions showing up on the brain in an MRI scan would certainly point in this direction. Objective evidence disclosed in a doctor's exam is key to any diagnosis. Two or more episodes lasting at least 24 hours and coming at least a month apart is considered to be an important indicator.

During this diagnostic period, Dr. Maitland explained the process to me. It is a matter of eliminating other possible diseases, one by one. "If we can't figure out what is wrong with you, then we tell you that you have multiple sclerosis," he said with a smile. As I continued to read, I discovered how true that really was. The several different tests that are used along with doctor-patient visits eliminate some diseases as possibilities. Many of the symptoms of MS are common symptoms of other diseases. A conclusive diagnosis is not at all a simple process.

The MRI is the best test to show the changes caused by MS. This can give clear evidence of scar tissue in deep parts of the brain and spinal cord that would indicate multiple sclerosis. When I had my first one, the person at the firm doing it said there was no indication of MS. A year later, the same thing happened.

During this time, and before diagnosis, I was home one evening reading a medical book that I had borrowed from a doctor friend of mine. As I often did when home by myself, I sat on the floor while reading. I was reading about different diseases and their symptoms when I came across the section on multiple sclerosis. As I read I knew, really knew, that I had MS.

I started laughing. I laughed so hard that I just rolled over on the floor holding my side. I know that is not the response to be expected from someone just learning that they have multiple sclerosis. For me, however, that knowledge was such a relief. For the first time since all of these strange things had been going on with my body, I knew that I did not have cancer; I had not had a stroke; and I did not have a tumor growing inside me. Racing through my mind was, "I only have multiple sclerosis. I can deal with that."

I was sitting on the floor feeling relieved when a "vision" flashed before me. I had recognized long before then that God often speaks through dreams and visions.

In my vision, I was in a one-room school house sitting on the floor with a friend. We looked to be eight or ten years old. The teacher was out of the room and we were chattering away. All of a sudden, the door opened and in walked our teacher. It was Jesus and he was carrying, not a two by four but, a four by four over one shoulder.

Without even pausing, he walked straight across the room to where we were sitting. He swung the four by four, hitting me solidly. The force of the swing sent me flying through the air. I slammed against the far wall before crumpling in a heap at the base of the wall. Without missing a step, he walked over to the wall, looked down, and very gently asked, "Now, will you pay attention?" I was reminded once again how important those daydreams or, night dreams, can be.

I knew I had MS; that my life had just taken a very sharp turn; and I was facing a real challenge.

My immediate challenge was to learn all I could about multiple sclerosis and how I could deal with it. That was the beginning of a real search for knowledge and a real battle to rebuild my body and reclaim my brain. It called for staying really focused and not losing sight of the objective – to heal myself. One of my all-time favorite sports figures, Yogi Berra, said it well, "You got to be careful if you don't know where you're going, because you might not get there."

Dr. Wray, a close friend for many years, asked me in the following years if I ever got depressed about having multiple sclerosis. He pointed out that it would not be uncommon. I could honestly say, "That has never depressed me."

I have always felt thankful that it wasn't something worse. Every time that I would see someone dealing with terrible health problems, I would know how really fortunate I was. It seemed that everywhere I turned, someone had problems bigger than mine. It still felt the same way years later, when my symptoms were so much worse. While it isn't a disease that kills, some people do die from complications they experience with MS.

At a later visit, Dr. Maitland told me that a spinal tap was about the only thing left for us to use as a diagnostic tool to conclusively diagnose. I said to him, "You know that I have MS and I know that I have MS. I don't see why I should suffer the discomfort that I will likely have from a spinal tap, just so you can say, "Yes, you have multiple sclerosis." He smiled and did not disagree, acknowledging that he wouldn't be doing anything differently if he knew that I had multiple sclerosis.

A year later, he scheduled another MRI. When the radiologist was out of town, Dr. Maitland asked them to send over the MRI so that he could read it. He asked them to also send over the MRI's that were taken the previous two years. All of them clearly showed the lesions (white spots) on my brain. For whatever reason, the radiologist had not concluded that I had multiple sclerosis.

I have never forgotten our next visit. He showed me the MRI's. My brain was completely covered with small white specks or plaque, which was scar tissue. The previous two MRI's looked exactly like the one that I had just taken. It had been obvious that I had multiple sclerosis when I first came to see him.

Now I had two major challenges facing me. First, I had to cope with the task of functioning in everyday life with a debilitating disease that promised to get worse. At the same time, I had to learn as much as I could about this disease, including what I needed to do to get through it. The task at hand seemed rather daunting, my biggest challenge yet.

Accepting responsibility for my health was not a matter of blame. Guilt never helps. At the most basic level, however, I knew that actions I had taken in my life had affected my health. If I had no responsibility for the disease then how could I expect to affect what it was doing to my body? It is really just as simple as knowing that eating too much and not exercising results in obesity, which causes various health problems. My illness was a wake-up call; a message to do things differently. The body sends the messages. It is up to us whether we listen.

My supervisor could not have been better. I would like to see the day when disabled people are all treated with the same compassion and helpfulness that he showed me. He was incredibly supportive and made numerous accommodations to keep me functioning and employed.

The parking system was based on seniority. My parking space was in a location that forced me to walk up a steep hill to get to our building. The steepness made it very difficult. The heat made it almost impossible. He was instrumental in the formulation of a rule that enabled me to park in the garage attached to the building because of my handicap.

He arranged for the department to install a computer at my house and I worked at home for a while. The department had a sick leave pool where all the members contributed hours from their sick leave to be used by members who required extended absences for illness. I exhausted my personal leave time, and had an extended period of leave provided by the sick leave pool.

All of this time, I continued to deteriorate, both physically and mentally. I finally reached a point that I was not really functional much of the time. My ability to concentrate was severely inhibited by what was going on with my body. My lack of short term memory, or recall, had made it increasingly more difficult to function as an attorney. I knew that.

This was a really scary experience for me. I knew it was time to go. I didn't know what would happen to me. I knew enough about the disease by then to know that things did not look good. At that point, I should have been more afraid than I was.

I ended up being unemployed for three years. For a while my condition continued to deteriorate before it started to get better. I learned a lot about being really dependent on other people; about living with a great deal of uncertainty every day of my life; and about how far one can go with a positive attitude and faith in God. Miracles happen. It wasn't about learning to do it by myself. It was about knowing that I had to do it. Sometimes help just materialized and sometimes I had to ask. I had help from family and friends for which I was grateful. I set about learning about the disease and I prayed.

The student is to select and evaluate facts.
The facts are locked up in the patient.
—Abraham Flexner

Chapter 3

Coming to the Mountain
(What is Multiple Sclerosis?)

Your body is perfect. It knows how to do all the things that bodies are capable of doing. It knows how to walk, sweat, sleep, be hungry, cry ... It's also a very good learner. You can teach it to swim, drive a car, write a letter, play a guitar, cut a diamond, or climb a mountain.
– Dr. Wayne Dyer

.   The body is capable of so much more than one might expect. It could be climbing a real mountain or, it could be doing it figuratively like fighting a serious disease.

Multiple sclerosis is an auto immune disease that attacks any area of the nervous system including the brain, the spinal cord and the optic nerve. In other words, the body's own immune system attacks its own tissues. This process destroys myelin, the fatty substance that coats and protects nerve fibers in the brain and spinal cord. Myelin acts like insulation on an electrical wire. It lets signals pass between different parts of the body, at high speed. Think about moving your toes and they move instantly -- that is fast! What happens with MS is a breakdown between the origination of the signal and its delivery.

The nerves underneath the myelin may also be damaged. Some symptoms and disabilities may repair themselves, while some may be permanent (see Chapter 6 on cognition). The immune system which normally helps fight against foreign invaders such as viruses and bacteria, now is triggered by something causing the body to attack itself. The cause of all this is still pure speculation. The truth is that no one knows why. This accounts for the many theories as to the underlying cause.

Some major hospitals and the National Multiple Sclerosis Society claim to know more than ever about Multiple Sclerosis, but researchers are still searching for its cause.

I heard this when I was diagnosed in the early nineties. I hear the same things said today. Very little has changed during that time.

The National Multiple Sclerosis Society has chapters all over the country. Many have a fundraiser called Walk MS. I read in a 2011 newsletter from a Chapter in Florida, "I have seen just how much Walk MS has changed the course of the disease ... in the last ten years. It's been amazing to witness the advancements in research ..." What total, unadulterated garbage! The pharmaceutical industry hasn't changed the course of the disease in the 19 years that have passed since I first saw my neurologist. The pharmaceuticals have made billions since then and don't offer one medication that even purports to cure the disease. This is discussed further in Chapter 9.

In an article from Mayo Clinic in 2010, I read that "doctors and researchers don't understand exactly why Multiple Sclerosis occurs in some people and not in others and that a combination of factors ranging from genetics to childhood infections may play a role." This was written in 2010 by someone at one of our nation's top hospitals. The same thing was true fifteen years ago. That is the actual status of our progress.

It was true in 1992, when I first went to see a neurologist about the strange things happening to me. It is true today, in 2011, as I am completing this book.

Many factors have been explored and several are considered to be possible contributors to the likelihood of someone having this disease. These include geography, age, gender, ethnic background, genetics, and infectious causes.

Some suspect that environmental factors trigger the disease in generally susceptible people. Because of my personal experience, this particular theory makes sense to me. Some patients have more than one person in their families with multiple sclerosis. This results in the theory that the risk is higher among those people who have a close blood relative with the disease. At the same time, many patients like myself, have no one in their families with the disease.

My siblings certainly had a similar environment growing up. But, environments changed as each sibling became an adult. If only genetics were involved, one of my four siblings would have been more likely to have the disease. Some theorize that the environment in the years through the age of fifteen is a factor affecting development of the disease. All of my siblings shared the same environment at those ages. By the time that I started exhibiting MS symptoms in my mid-forties, I had twenty-five years of environmental factors which were not all the same as my siblings. So, who knows? Is the propensity to have the disease established early? Are the environmental factors in those years the important ones?

Between two and three million people around the world are thought to have multiple sclerosis. Over four hundred thousand people in the United States have been diagnosed. Women seem to get the disease at a rate about two or three times greater than that of men. I am not aware that anyone knows why.

Most people that are diagnosed seem to be between twenty and fifty years old. People in northern Europe and in the northern United States seem to get it at a greater rate than in the southern parts of both continents.

People from many different backgrounds seem to get the disease. The disease is not considered to be contagious. Some think it is triggered by an infection, like a virus. This trigger, it is thought, activates a type of white blood cell which starts a process that attacks and damages the nerve cells in the central nervous system.

Studies of migration patterns have shown that people born in an area of the world with a high risk of multiple sclerosis who then move to an area with a lower risk before the age of fifteen acquire the risk of their new area. Who is to say how reliable these studies are? Why the age of fifteen is considered important is not really known.

Some of the data suggest that exposure to some environmental agent that occurs before puberty may predispose a person to develop multiple sclerosis later on. Some people think the reason may have something to do with vitamin D, which the body produces naturally when exposed to enough sun. People who live closer to the equator are exposed to greater amounts of sunlight year round. They tend to have higher levels of naturally produced vitamin D. This is thought to have a beneficial impact on immune function and may help protect against autoimmune diseases like multiple sclerosis. This possible relationship has been investigated for a long period of time.

Scientists continue to look at multiple sclerosis clusters. These are higher than expected numbers of cases of MS that have occurred over a specific time period in a certain area. This may provide clues to different factors that are involved such as the environment, toxins, diet or trace metal exposures. Any of these may cause or trigger the disease. There has been no clear answer.

Viruses possibly cause demyelination and inflammation and may be a triggering factor in multiple sclerosis. More than a dozen viruses including measles, canine distemper, human herpes virus 6, Epstein Barr, chlamydia and pneumonia have been investigated to determine if they are involved in the development of MS. None have proven to be connected.

We know that disruption of energy flow caused by the damaged myelin results in a wide variety of symptoms and combinations. I am not aware of any disease with more potential symptoms than multiple sclerosis. There are 40-50 different ones. Patients don't have all of them. You can imagine the number of potential combinations that are possible. In my nineteen years of getting acquainted with the disease, I have never known of two patients with exactly the same combination of symptoms. If I named all of mine, of which I was aware, there would probably be more than a dozen.

In addition to the different combinations that are possible, very few of these symptoms are unique to multiple sclerosis. This makes diagnosis very difficult. Having one or several of the symptoms does not mean you have MS. It may be something else. The many symptoms have been categorized into different groupings ... visual, motor, sensory, coordination and balance, bowel, bladder and sexual, cognitive, and others. I won't attempt to list or discuss them all! They are not that difficult to find.

The effect to the legs is a very noticeable example. Multiple sclerosis may be causing the problem, or it may be something else. As the disease progresses, walking becomes more difficult. Use of a walking cane sometimes is necessary. I used one for several years. To begin with, I needed it to steady myself as I walked. Eventually, as my walking improved, I carried it "just in case." While I didn't like drawing attention to my disability, sometimes I was fortunate I had the cane. It did assist me in maintaining my balance. Eventually, after I no longer needed it, I came to think it was quite debonair.

I went through similar phases with the handicapped placard for my car. For a long time, I simply resisted thinking of myself as handicapped. To the most casual observer, I obviously was. The heat finally did it. As I would walk across a parking lot in this northwest Florida summer heat, I would struggle. It slowly dawned on me. I needed to get a handicapped placard for my car. Theoretically, I could park near the entrance of the mall or office building in a reserved parking space.

One of my earlier symptoms was the slurring of words. A problem with speech is not unusual. It became progressively worse in my early years of MS. At the time of my three year break from employment, I was having difficulty communicating.

I saw a speech therapist for almost a year. She was truly a guardian angel. When I began seeing her, I had great difficulty speaking clearly. I would do different voice exercises in her office. At home, I would sit on my floor and repeat over and over, "How now, brown cow." It was a slow process but my enunciation improved tremendously. She literally taught me to talk again. People have commented on how slowly and distinctly that I talk sometimes. That came from my many hours of speech therapy – some with her and some unsupervised.

During that time, she became my "life coach" as well as my speech therapist. A couple of small, but scary, things happened. I left an egg boiling on the stove. The water boiled out of the pot and by the time the egg exploded, the metal pot had a hole in it. Egg was hanging from the ceiling and the walls. Another day, I left the water running in the bath tub. I remembered it when I felt water in my living room carpet. The whole place was flooded.

The results in each case could have been much worse. A friend came and vacuumed the water out of my carpets. I cleaned the "exploded egg" from the walls and ceilings of my kitchen. I was really embarrassed each time.

My speech therapist assisted me in setting up some rules to avoid those things happening again. They were simple. If I had water running in the tub, I had to sit there until I turned the water off. If I had something on the stove cooking, I had to sit there until I turned off the stove.

Her husband was a sports writer and they moved from Tallahassee a short time later.

Many times I have wanted to thank her. I hope she will see this and know how much I appreciate her.

For a long time, governments and businesses were slow to provide handicapped spaces. It amazes me to see remaining resistance to providing adequate parking, or other reasonable accommodations. After my three years of not being employed, I worked for a state agency that always seemed to resist providing basic accommodations to the handicapped.

While working in the agency's Office of the Inspector General I got a "close up" view of many attitudes toward the handicapped. It wasn't just a matter of not having sufficient parking spaces. The agency resisted making very basic accommodations necessary for people to perform their jobs. It was obvious things such as not having proper curb cuts at convenient locations so that a person in a wheelchair could make it to the sidewalk. The agency did not insure elevator lights worked properly so that a deaf person could "see" what floor we were on. Or, not having the bells working so that a blind person could "hear" what floor we were on. The agency failed to recognize, or accept, that a given task might take longer for a disabled person.

I worked under four different Inspectors General. Three of the four were outstanding in complying with the intent of the law. As in the rest of the work force, attitudes and opinions about disabilities varied from ensuring the disabled person succeeded to expecting the disabled person to perform every task as if he/she was not disabled.

Looking back, I am still amazed at the attitude displayed by some people. When faced with a situation needing attention, their first thought was how to avoid accommodating a disabled person. They would sit there and argue that the state agency didn't have responsibility under the Americans with Disabilities Act (ADA). Even when a solution was simple and obvious, management and their attorneys would often look for a justification *not* to do anything. Some of those people are still there in high level positions. One Inspector General would just speak to the people involved and resolve the problems. This was more efficient than being stalled by top management who insisted the law did not apply to them.

Helping the handicapped is not always a top priority. This is true at every level. While our government promoted war in the Middle East, the treatment of wounded and disabled soldiers at Walter Reed Hospital in Bethesda fell to scandalous levels. The soldiers who were wounded and disabled while fighting in our wars were obviously not a priority.

Primary symptoms of MS are the direct result of damage to the myelin and nerve fibers in the central nervous system. Secondary symptoms are the complications that may arise as a result of the primary symptoms. For example, inactivity can result in less muscle tone and disuse weakness, not related to demyelination. Poor postural alignment and trunk control may directly result from inactivity rather than from the disease itself. Likewise, decreased bone density and resulting increased risk of falling may result from inactivity rather than from the multiple sclerosis that precipitated it.

For a long time, exposure to heat was very disabling to me. I could not be out in the sun for very long. I could not take a hot bath, and that went on for years. That actually was one of the first things I noticed in the early stages of my MS. I had always loved taking a hot bath. At a time when I had not yet been diagnosed, I had trouble getting out of the bathtub. I felt weak and unstable. It took me a while to make the connection to heat. It really wasn't until after I had been diagnosed and had begun researching the disease that I remembered what a problem sitting in hot water had become for me.

Numbness in MS patients is one of the more common symptoms of the disease, although I did not experience it. It is among the first symptoms noticed or reported by many. This numbness may appear in any of the extremities. It may vary from a small spot on the end of the thumb to an entire leg. Very often, it is the extremities such as fingers and toes that are most affected. It may be acute or chronic. It can last for a few hours, and then return to normal. It can last for days or even weeks. If only a small section of the arm, or a finger, is involved, it may not be a big problem. When a large body part like a leg is affected, it may seriously affect one's quality of life, at the workplace and at home.

For patients with advanced multiple sclerosis, numbness of the face can be more serious. Patients may bite the inside of their mouths when eating, or burn themselves with hot food. Fire and hot water can produce serious burns anywhere that heat cannot be felt. They may not immediately be aware of this because of the numbness. Open wounds inside of the mouth may cause no pain, but become seriously infected before the patient notices. It is extremely important that patients with numbness around the mouth area check regularly for cuts and burns.

Many sufferers of multiple sclerosis experience other abnormal sensations on a daily basis. Sometimes the numbness alternates with a tingling sensation. Most of the day an area might be numb and then suddenly come alive with "pins and needles." This may be because sensory messages from the brain to the affected area reach their destination for a period of time and then they no longer get through and the area goes numb again.

A common symptom is spasticity. This refers to feelings of muscle stiffness and a wide range of involuntary muscle spasms. It is thought to affect about eighty percent of people with multiple sclerosis to some degree. Sudden movements, extreme temperatures and humidity, infections and even tight clothing are all thought to be possible triggers of spasticity.

Massages are highly recommended to treat this symptom and can really assist in increasing comfort and range of motion. They were really great for me, at times.

Looking at my eyes directly in front of you, you would not have noticed a particular problem of mine. But, moving my eyes from side to side might disclose a problem to an observant person watching them.

When I would cut my eyes to one side, and then return them to straight ahead, the eyes would not follow the same track. One eye would move faster than the other, and have a "flutter."

While loss of sight for some period of time often happens with multiple sclerosis, only once did I experience that. I don't even know that it was MS that caused the loss of sight. I was returning home from church. As I walked into my house, I lost my vision. Everything in both eyes went dark. I could see "light" where each window was. I couldn't make out any forms, just light from the windows.

I will never forget the panic I felt. I stood there for a few minutes pondering what to do. I decided that I was tired and would just go to sleep. I felt my way back to my bedroom, which was fairly simple since it was something that I did every day.

I slowly walked into my bedroom, always touching the wall, and then the dresser, to keep my bearings. Then I touched the bed, turned around and sat, and pulled off my shoes. I lay down and soon went to sleep. Rarely have I had trouble sleeping, no matter what was going on. This was no exception. I slept for several hours.

When I woke and opened my eyes, I could see perfectly. That never happened again.

Symptoms may include changes in sensation or muscle weakness. People have muscle spasms in varying degrees. They may simply be irritating or they may be very disabling. Some patients have problems with coordination and balance. This may be seen as a progressive type of symptom and get gradually worse as time goes by. It can become difficult to move around. This symptom is common.

I learned that I had to be more careful about lots of things. Falls, bumps, and accidents can lead to broken bones. Things that had always been second nature to me, no longer were. I was unpacking some boxes and putting the contents where they belonged. I lost my balance and fell backward into a box. I was on my back in the box, with my hands and feet sticking straight up in the air. I could not move. I started laughing at my predicament, thinking about how I must look. Eventually, I managed to rock the box from side to side until it turned over. From there, I managed to slowly inch myself out of the box.

A short time later, unpacking those same boxes, I managed to wedge one foot between two of them. When I turned, that foot did not turn with me and my ankle was severely sprained.

My worst fall came after my MS symptoms had pretty much disappeared and had little to do with my multiple sclerosis. I had just finished a six mile walk and was within a block of my house. I failed to see a hole because it was full of grass. When I stepped in it, I just pitched forward. My face broke my fall and was so swollen that I went to see a doctor. Fortunately, there was no bleeding. After being assured by a doctor that the swelling (my eye was shut) was just air, I punctured it and gently squeezed out the air and the "swelling" was gone.

Another time I was in a hurry coming down my stairs. About four steps from the bottom, I caught my heel and pitched forward. That was a long, hard fall. I didn't break anything, but I was sore and stiff for days.

Fatigue is a very common symptom and one that bothered me for years in my journey with multiple sclerosis. This is discussed at greater length in Chapter 8.

I have known of people complaining of pain, sometimes acute, but this has rarely been an issue for me. There were times that I hurt, but my pain was more of an aching feeling, with one extremely important exception. Many years ago, I had trigeminal neuralgia. I intend to cover that in another book, along with some other medical problems that I have faced on my journey. A recent experience with it seriously delayed completion of this book and prompted me to address it now.

In places it is listed as a symptom of multiple sclerosis because the vast majority of people who have it also have MS. In places it is listed as a separate disease and some patients who have it don't have MS. Clearly, it seems to me, it is not a symptom of multiple sclerosis, but a disease itself. Some people experience both.

Trigeminal neuralgia is one of the most painful diseases known. It involves crippling, shock-like, stabbing pain in the face. Usually it is on one side, but can be on both. The name comes from the name of the affected nerve, trigeminal, and from the word neuralgia which means a severe, stabbing pain often related to a nerve.

Ordinary stimuli such as touch, talking, eating, or the lightest touching of the face may cause intense, burning, electric, shock-like pain which may last a few seconds or several minutes. The pain may come a few times an hour or several times a minute. Many authorities believe that compression of the trigeminal nerve by a vein or an artery is the main cause. Direct injury to that nerve may also cause an attack. Five to ten percent of MS patients experience trigeminal neuralgia. As many as ten percent of trigeminal neuralgia patients don't have multiple sclerosis.

The first time I had trigeminal neuralgia many years ago, my neurologist put me on medication. He told me, accurately, that it might take six months to stop the pain. It did. He also said that I would need to take it the rest of my life unless I wanted to re-experience the pain. I stopped it a few years later, with his knowledge, as I was reducing my intake of prescription meds in general.

An acupuncturist told me he could stop the pain if it came back, and he did. His name is Kerry Abaco, Doctor of Oriental Medicine. He recently relocated to Panama City, Florida, after which I had the most painful resurgence of my trigeminal neuralgia in years. The pain was so intense that I could not write for two weeks. On a trip he was making to Tallahassee, he called and arranged to meet me. He gave me a one-hour treatment. My pain disappeared. I am back to my writing.

For most people, symptoms of multiple sclerosis appear sporadically, coming in episodes called relapses or exacerbations or flare-ups. Often, this is a very gradual progression, as the symptoms become more troublesome.

Multiple sclerosis relapses are very unpredictable, coming with little notice. One of many unknown things about the disease is that the relapse rate among pregnant women seems to be significantly lower than among the general population of women with the disease. While this has been observed for many years, no one knows why.

All of this is to say, again, that people with multiple sclerosis have varying symptoms in many different combinations. Some people have minor irritants. Others have symptoms that are very debilitating. Some cover short periods of time, while some cover long periods.

Sometimes what seems to be a negative incident may well be an anonymous visitation from a higher power.
-- Bernie S. Siegel, M.D.

Chapter 4

Looking Back
(My Background)

All of the stuff in your life has arrived to serve you rather than to make you a servant of the stuff.   -- Dr. Wayne Dyer

Opinions about the causes of multiple sclerosis are still very diverse, involving much guesswork. No one knows. One theory is that a propensity for the disease is there, and may be "triggered" by different environmental factors. MS may not make itself known until much later (ages 20-50), but many professionals believe the groundwork is in place by the mid-teens. For this reason, it is important to include the story of my growing up.

My early years were filled with stress. A big part of that was because I grew up in Northwest Florida, known as the "Florida Panhandle." This was one of the poorest areas of the state. Today Florida still ranks fiftieth in per capita spending on education. It was ravaged by the depression and still in the early days of recovery. It was totally dependent on farming. It was the "Florida frontier" and still is the real Florida to me. This rural area of Florida is not the same vacation destination that most vacationers visit.

Times were really tough but we had food to eat. We had shelter when it rained and we had a wood burning fireplace when it was cold; sometimes brutally cold. We rarely saw snow but the ground was so cold that sometimes it was frozen. Some days it would never thaw. There were cracks in the floor of our house big enough to see the ground underneath and the chickens scratching for food.

I remember when electricity first came through our area. Daddy paid an "electrician" twenty-five dollars to wire our house. Before that we had kerosene lamps and the fireplace to provide light. A covered wagon pulled by mules came by once a week. From this rolling store we purchased essentials such as flour, sugar, salt, and other items we did not produce. We paid for these necessities with things we produced, such as eggs, butter and canned vegetables.

Farming was still done with mules and I learned how to plow when I was nine years old. Daddy knew he didn't have the patience to teach me and hired a man who lived nearby to do that. After one day of instruction without destroying too much of the crop, I was plowing on my own. Our first tractor came years later along with a used pickup truck. By my junior year in high school we owned a used car.

Everything about my years growing up was stressful. Some of the stress was created simply by the hard times in which we grew up. Most of it came from my father, who was both an alcoholic and a workaholic. Both had a lasting effect on me and my life.

My daddy's mother was a single mom. She raised eight children by herself in the depression. Her husband spent many years in prison for abusing his oldest daughter, Daddy's sister. My grandmother, Mama Blanche to us, turned him in and testified for the prosecution at his trial. She was a strong woman.

My father was only six at the time that happened. It shaped much of his life. I think the shame just consumed him. He hated his father, never forgiving him for what he did. He rarely ever mentioned him.

I learned later that living in the past is not healthy for anyone. Today is all we have. Ideally we will learn from our experiences, good and bad, and move on.

It is essential to understand the importance of forgiveness. Not forgiving someone for a hurt they have caused you or someone else can do great damage – not to that person but to you, and those around you. I discuss this because it is a significant part of my story and had a real impact on my life. You can't change what was done to you. But you do control your treatment of others. You have the power to forgive. I forgave my dad eventually and it wasn't easy. My inability to forgive him, hurt me not him

Dad was one of the angriest, most bitter people that I have ever known. He was not able to forgive and that colored his whole life. As is often the case, the ones he hurt the most were the ones closest to him, his family.

When I was only a few years old, I heard a knock at the door. Daddy went to answer it. Like most kids that age, I was curious and "tagged" along to see who was there.

It was a neighbor. He said, "Roy, I just wanted to let you know that your daddy died." Dad responded, "I don't have a daddy," and closed the door in his face. He never said a word to us about the man at the door, then or later.

Some of my most vivid memories of those years involved Dad's drinking episodes. He was a mean, angry drunk. He was abusive to anyone who got in his way, especially my mom. One night (I must have been four or five) he was on the front porch shooting at the chickens in the barnyard because "they were making too much noise." Mom was attempting, unsuccessfully, to get him to come inside. When I think about that, I am reminded of a question that I read somewhere, "Who is the more irrational? The drunk, or the sober person trying to reason with him?" Years later, Mom and I have laughed about that.

From early elementary school until after I left, he didn't drink. Nonetheless, that anger we saw when he was drunk always seemed to boil just below the surface. When I was about ten I laid my bicycle, my most prized possession, on the ground in front of his truck. He ran over my bike and it was crushed. I was horrified. Instead of consoling me, he took off his belt. He gave me a brutal beating, with Mom begging him to stop. I still remember lying on the bed crying while Mom "doctored" my back. The next day my shirt had blood in a couple of places from where his beating had broken the skin.

That incident with the bike was not the first time that I had experienced his brutality. When I was about six I witnessed him slap my mom in the face. If my brother Jerry, almost two years older, had not picked up a stick and stepped in front of her, I don't know what would have happened. The sight of this little person with his stick stopped him. He went in the house.

Of course, he never hesitated to use his belt on us. I received severe whippings with it all the way up to my high school years. For fighting, arguing, 'talking back," or whatever he was upset about. How logical was that? His punishment for us for fighting with each other was to take off his belt and beat us, and I don't mean two or three taps. Of course, it fit perfectly with his often repeated instructions to "Do as I say, not as I do."

We were probably six or so when we started working in the fields. Until then, it was household chores, which continued as long as we were home because Mom spent so much time in the fields and the garden. I remember Jerry, at five or six, standing in a chair to wash dishes because he wasn't tall enough to reach the dish pan.

Milking the cow was one of the many chores that had to be done before school. The chickens and hogs had to be fed. Eggs had to be collected from the hen house.

Inside, dishes had to be washed. Beds had to be made. Floors had to be swept. If you had been doing barnyard chores, you had to take a bath again. We didn't have running water until I was in junior high school. What we had was cold water in a wash tub warmed with water heated on a stove. When it was winter and freezing outside, a sponge bath had to suffice.

While we were doing morning chores, mom was already in the field working, or in the garden, or making our clothes, or quilting, etc. She had made breakfast for us before we did chores.

We had to be dressed and ready for the school bus by seven. When it was freezing outside, we might stand in that cold, bundled up, for 15 or 20 minutes. For the driver to stay on schedule, we had to wait by the road. We did not dare miss the bus, and the driver would not wait. You were either by the highway or he didn't stop.

It was the same coming home. When school was out, we went to our bus and loaded for the trip home. If we weren't on the bus, we were left. That happened only once. I was in the first grade and my brother was two years older. For some reason, we didn't make it to the bus fast enough that afternoon and the bus left without us.

When we realized the bus had left, we started running. From the school to the edge of town was a couple of miles. We were well outside of town, still running, when a man on a truck stopped and got out. Very kindly, he asked who we were and where we were going. He recognized our names and knew we were several miles from home. He put us in his truck and told us that he knew where we lived and took us home.

He told my parents where he found us. Not a lot of people, including us, had automobiles in northwest Florida at that time. We were fortunate to get a ride. I was afraid of what Daddy was going to do to us for missing the bus, and I could sense his anger. His anger, however, was not directed toward us. Although the bus driver lived several miles away, my dad started walking. I was asleep when he got home and I never knew what was said, or what happened. I am sure it wasn't pleasant. In all the years that followed, no bus driver ever left one of us again.

It is amazing, really, that we didn't suffer more serious injuries than we did. I broke a collar bone when I fell while running through the house to see a road grader that I heard coming. At the time, engines of any kind were not that common. I was about six when that happened. I still remember going to the doctor and being bandaged.

My youngest brother chopped another younger brother in the head with a garden hoe. Blood was gushing from his head when my dad ran to him to see what the screaming was about. Both brothers were only a few years old at the time. My dad, in an effort to calm him, said, "He didn't mean to do it." My youngest brother, who had done the chopping, said, "Oh, yes I did too; he was taking my dirt."

Another time we were playing at my grandparents who lived about a quarter of a mile down the road. They kept their mule in a pasture behind their barn and we decided to ride him. We were taking turns and my youngest brother was on the mule. This mule was stubborn, as mules are prone to be. He decided he was finished giving us rides and headed for the barn. The barn had a tin roof and that part of the barn was high enough for the mule to go under but not high enough for the rider. The tin roof would have cut his chest.

Fortunately, my brother realized this. Just before the mule reached the barn, he slid off. He hit the ground on his side and dislocated an elbow.

Years later when I saw Michael Jordan jump and hang in the air just before dunking a basketball, I was reminded of an afternoon when I was running through the woods. I wasn't more than ten or twelve. Running along a trail, I saw a puddle ahead. I didn't slow down, intending to jump it. In mid-air, I saw a large moccasin sunning on the other side of the puddle. I would be landing right on top of him and I knew their reputation well. I seemed to freeze, suspended in mid-air. It was as if the snake saw me and slithered off into the bushes as I landed where it had been.

When Daddy was younger he was a very controlling person. He thrived on being the authoritarian. In the words of a brother, Dad was an absolute "control freak" with us and with our mother.

During the first couple of years they were married they moved several times. They lived in Tennessee, Georgia, and Florida as he held numerous jobs. To Mom, it was always "I'm going to wherever. You can come if you want to."

He wasn't satisfied with controlling what we did. He was determined to control what we thought. He was controlling and demanding to the point of being abusive. The emotional abuse was often worse than the beatings.

He didn't want us reading during the day. "If that is all you have to do, I will find something for you to do." He also wanted to control what we read. If he caught me reading something that he didn't like, he would take the book and burn it. That would follow the stern lecture about the "trash" I was reading. Anything about politics or social issues was really "asking for trouble."

I would crawl under the house and read so he would not catch me reading something that met with his disapproval. It could be a novel, non-fiction, or a newspaper. It didn't matter. My grandmother Blackburn, Mom's mother, always subscribed to the Atlanta Constitution. When she finished it, she passed it on to us, so I grew up reading it. For a long time that was our "window to the outside world."

We didn't have air conditioning in those early years. Often, it was too hot at night to sleep. I was conscious of the perspiration rolling off my body as I tossed and turned. During the day, the dirt would burn my feet as I often worked without shoes.

Swimming in the creek a few miles from the house provided occasional relief. The running water in the creek was always cold. We looked forward to those trips. One day, some neighbor boys had tied a long rope to a tree limb in a large oak tree hanging over the creek. Several feet up the bank, they constructed a platform several feet high where they would stand. Holding the rope, they would swing out over the creek. They would reach a height of 15 to 20 feet above the water before releasing the rope and diving into the water below.

It was beautiful and looked like so much fun. I had to try it. I climbed onto the platform and grabbed the rope. Not knowing any better, I had my arms bent at the elbow. I started this beautiful arc downward toward the water. As I reached the bottom of the arc, the weight of my body and its downward motion snapped my elbows straight with such force that the rope was torn from my hands. I hit the bank instead of the water and was fortunate to have no injuries. The wind was knocked from me.

A boy that I didn't know was not so lucky. He swung out over the creek. When he released the rope and dove, he was not over the deeper part of the creek. Traveling head first, he hit the bottom of the creek and broke his neck, paralyzing him from the neck down.

Even with all the tragedy, there was sometimes a bit of humor. I have laughed many times at my memories of milking the cow. Usually, we gave her some hay to eat while we were milking. That would involve sitting on my heels, with the bucket in the left hand while my right hand gently squeezed milk from each udder. By the time I finished, I would usually have a gallon, or so, of milk in the bucket.

While I was milking, I was constantly avoiding the flies and the cow's long tail. She swished it to chase flies landing on her. The floor of the stall would be covered with dried cow manure, covered with a blanket of hay. Then rain would run through the barn leaving a soggy, dirty floor of cow manure. One day, after a heavy rain, a bug stung the cow. She kicked, knocking me backward into the dirty cow manure. I dropped the milk pail as she planted her dirty hoof in my bucket of milk. I have laughed many times thinking about that. While some of these events are funny to me now, most are not!!

The annual grind would start every winter. When it was cold a hog would be slaughtered and later a cow. The neighbors would help and each would take enough meat home to make a meal.

Everyone had a two week break from school for the Christmas holidays. Our break was to spend hours working in the fields where another ten acres had been cleared. We would be picking up roots and piling them to burn. Sometimes it would freeze. We would have to keep a fire going to avoid frostbite.

Watermelons would be planted in February or March. One year, he guessed that the winter would be over early, but he guessed wrong. The watermelon plants were up and growing when a late, unexpected freeze was on its way. Daddy took us all out of school at lunchtime.

Using pages from old *Sears* catalogs and farm magazines, we covered every plant in a ten acre field that afternoon. We covered each plant with a page and put dirt on the corners to keep it from blowing away. The next day after school, we uncovered all of the plants. The end result was that we had the earliest watermelons on the market in our area. This made for a really profitable year.

The plants would grow into large vines covering the entire ground. Plants would bloom and the blooms would turn into melons, tiny at first. As the melons grew, they would ripen in the sun. The melons would be twenty-five or thirty pounds and sometimes even larger.

I have always remembered overhearing a conversation about Daddy at the local store, "That Roy is the luckiest man alive when it comes to planting at the right time." The truth is that I never knew a farmer who worked longer and harder, and smarter, than Daddy did.

Mom worked even harder than he did. She worked in the fields with us. She had a huge garden with a great variety of vegetables. She was the best cook I have ever known. We ate her canned vegetables year round. She spent hours "canning" vegetables and later preparing them for the freezer. Not to mention preparing three meals a day. She made our clothes, kept house, and helped with our homework. Somehow she managed to provide us with the only affection we had.

When the melons were ripe, my dad would walk through the field clipping the stems on ripened melons. We would follow behind, carrying the melons which he "clipped" from the vines, to the nearest road.

We would go through the entire field, usually about ten acres, and have all of the roads lined with melons. We created the roads by moving the vines between two rows in opposite directions when the melons were still nothing but blooms. Then we would drive the tractor, pulling a trailer, down the road with melons lining each side. One person would drive the tractor; one person would stand in the trailer; and one person would stand on each side of the trailer.

As the trailer slowly moved along, the two people on the ground would "toss" the melons to the person in the trailer. The work was fast and back breaking.

We would get a short break of ten to twenty minutes when the loaded trailer was being pulled to the truck. Then we would go to work moving the melons from the trailer to the truck which would be taking them to market in New Orleans, Montgomery or Birmingham. Daddy might be gone overnight or he might be gone for two or three days.

Sometimes, he would take one of us with him. I made one trip. Those trips were long and tiresome. I preferred being at home and getting some much needed rest. The pressure was not as intense when he was gone, although he always left us with more work to do than we could get done.

I have vivid memories of one of the longest, hardest periods of work that I ever endured, on the farm, or since. It came at a time that we actually had a chance for some relief from the constant financial pressure under which we lived.

Daddy had the hardest working bunch of "slaves" that I ever saw, starting with Mom, to do his bidding. This involved non-stop stress for the whole family. It included working hours that were abusive for adults and certainly for pre-teens and teenagers. All of us were expected to excel in school although we worked long hours when we got home. We were allowed almost no social life outside of school while growing up.

Even when prospering, we were always "land poor." Everything we had was tied up in land, with little for anything else. The stress was extreme … from my earliest memories, all the way through high school. Daddy always made certain of that.

We had been debt free for a short period of time and had enough money to live for the next year. Daddy had a chance to buy an additional forty acres joining the backside of our farm. He got a three year loan from the owner/seller to buy the forty acres. He could have gotten bank loans with better terms but didn't. I remember once he thought he might need one and went to check it out. They would have loaned him whatever he needed. He had land, no debt, and a series of successful years farming. He was the perfect borrower.

We had a family meeting to discuss buying the land. It was the only such meeting I recall ever having about anything. Normally, he just did whatever he wanted to do. Our job was to do as we were told.

He knew we had all been under incredible stress for years and, now, had a chance to jointly catch our breaths. But he wanted the land. This charade was to make it appear that it was a family decision to do what he was going to do anyway. Mom had not been excited with the idea. She knew we all needed some down time. The "family meeting" was to stifle her objections.

That first year, we cleared about ten acres of the newly acquired forty acre tract. Then our hard work started – picking up roots. Sometimes it was so cold we could only pick up the roots for a few minutes and then warm our hands by the fire. On the really cold days, this would go on all day. Eventually, there would be no roots left.

Later, the watermelon plants were growing and Daddy was plowing to keep down the weeds. He came home at lunch one day really discouraged. He had detected some type of disease on the plants, even though they were small. He knew that the disease would spread by the time the melons had time to grow. Some types of disease would get on the melons themselves, eating away at the outside covering of the melons called rinds, and they would not be marketable.

He considered plowing them under and planting something else. Instead, he left the melon plants growing and finished plowing them.

Normally, harvesting the melons would last a month or more. As melons were removed from the vines, smaller ones would grow larger. Toward the end of the growing season, ripe melons might weigh no more than ten or fifteen pounds and we were still selling them. We might only be getting ten or fifteen cents per melon. Today, this size melon sells for $8.00 at the local grocery store. Some years, someone would come along toward the end and buy everything left in the field for a lump sum price. The buyer harvested those without any help from us.

The crop that particular year grew fast. The disease covered the vines but never affected the melons. No sores ever developed on them as he had expected. Normally, new melons would keep coming on the plants. Harvesting would last a few weeks. That year, it was fast and furious. We worked for ten straight days, including Sunday, getting to the field by five or six in the morning. We would work at getting them out of the field during the day and loading the trucks until midnight. There was a large security light where the truck was parked. We could see how to load the melons that we had spent all day hauling out of the field and stacking in the shade of a large oak tree. We survived on four or five hours of sleep each day, doing some of the hardest work that I had ever done.

We never had a better melon crop than we had that year. We paid for the entire forty acres with that one crop of watermelons. The stress from that hard work did not even approach the level of stress to which we were normally subjected. During these ten days we were busy and under his complete control. He didn't subject us to his usual mental torture.

Before we started harvesting watermelons, the other crops were already planted and growing. That had been done after the melons were planted.

Daddy would joke about how educated he was. He left school in the tenth grade. The truth is that he was really "bright." As was my mom who had been valedictorian of her class. He would study farm magazines, *The Progressive Farmer*, *The Farm Journal*, and the *Almanac*. He would then make an educated guess as to the best times to plant the various crops each year. Those decisions were always important. Replanting could cost a lot of money as well as time. Seed and fertilizer were both expensive. An entire crop could be lost to weather conditions. I remember droughts that lasted so long that we had to haul water, by mule and wagon, from a creek miles away to keep the livestock alive.

He paid close attention to weather forecasts. From the almanac and farm magazines for long term predictions. The radio, and later the television were for daily updates. He studied and learned the newest seeds available; what kind and how much fertilizer to use for good crops and to avoid depleting the soil; and how to rotate his crops effectively and maximize production. For example, after the melons were raised on the recently cleared fields, it would be used for pasture for a while and later for other crops. By this time, he would have discovered some water source. It might be a stream or he would hire someone with a bulldozer to excavate a pond and build a dam, if needed.

As a taskmaster, Dad was at his toughest in the fields. Many times, I worked all day pulling weeds from the peanuts, only to get a totally negative reaction from him the next morning when he came to check our work.

In the early morning, when the dew still covered everything, the leaves on the peanuts looked very different from the leaves on the plants that we called a coffee weed. Later in the day, when the sunlight dried everything, you could hardly tell the difference. It was easy to miss the weeds if they were not taller than the peanut vines.

He knew that, but didn't share that part with us. His purpose in not doing so was to justify telling us to spend another day redoing what we had done the day before. We always had the cleanest crops.

About the same time the cotton plants were growing we would have to "chop cotton." The rows would have a continuous row of little plants. That was to make sure we had a crop. Then we would go along with hoes and "chop" some plants so the remaining plants would have room to grow.

His objective was to keep us busy all of the time, and always trying harder. To him, he was being a good father. He knew what kind of mischief he would have been in and assumed we would do the same. He had to keep us busy every single day, "for our own good." This attitude from him was constant the entire time we were growing up. It didn't matter that we were good students, didn't get into any real trouble, and always worked hard.

In between planting, cultivating, and harvesting he would find other jobs for us. Some because they needed to be done and some just to keep us busy. Neighboring farmers would hire us because we were hard workers. We got the money and he kept us busy. No rest for us. Only when it was raining were we allowed to rest.

One "make work" job was to have us clean fence rows with weed slings and garden hoes and axes. We had wire fences crisscrossing the entire farm. This was primarily to keep livestock, whether ours or someone else's, from roaming over the farm eating the crops. They might be in a pasture and well fed but, given the opportunity, they would go in another field and ravage whatever crop was there.

Some people don't know peanuts are part of the root system. Like other plants they get a significant portion of their nourishment from the green plant above the ground. When cows had the chance, they would eat that green part of the plant. Hogs would "root out" the peanuts from under the ground and eat them. Both would get through the fences (over, under, or through) and lay waste to a beautiful field of peanuts or corn.

Most farmers didn't bother keeping their fence rows clean. Weeds would grow, making the fences look more impenetrable to the livestock. It didn't necessarily look bad, and did no discernible damage to the crops, no matter how thick the vegetation along the fence was.

There were reasons why the grown-over fence rows were useful. Insects helped to pollinate crops and lived in those fence rows. Birds, such as quail, had their nests there and hatched their eggs in them. None of that mattered to my dad. We had the cleanest fence rows in the whole county, as well as the cleanest crops. More importantly, we didn't have time for "mischief."

This took its toll on each of us. I would bring home a report card with an A in every subject. He would look at my report card and say, sometimes with a twinkle in his eye, "Is this the best you can do?" The grades would be numerical but in the "A" range. It was sometimes humorous, but always with the message that nothing was ever good enough. For citizenship, everyone would get an "S" for satisfactory or a "U" for unsatisfactory. We would always be chastised by him for "only" getting satisfactory.

We always had a garden and grew most of our food on the farm. During what we called canning season, spring and summer, we would spend hours shelling beans and peas, peeling tomatoes, and cleaning corn. During the early years, we canned them in quart jars and later we had a freezer that we filled with containers of fresh vegetables. We always had plenty to eat and Mom was a great cook. I think my favorite dish was a tomato sauce. It was made with tomatoes, onions, peppers and spices. We ate it on meats and on vegetables. It gave everything that tangy, spicy flavor.

Eating was such a treat, and caused me such problems at the same time. When we were busy all the time, it wasn't a problem. After having been overweight most of my younger life, I was trim by the time I was a senior in high school. Working outside in that heat burns a lot of calories.

After watermelons the next crop to be harvested was peanuts. In the early days, the first part of the process was simply to plow them. This was done with a plow blade which went under the plant including the roots and just rolled it over, exposing the nuts. They would sit for a few days as the sun dried out the dirt on the peanuts. Then, by hand, we would pick up the plants and shake them, getting rid of all the dirt. Next we would do what was called "stacking" peanuts. We would dig a hole and put in a pole which would stick about eight or nine feet out of the ground. Then, about a foot off the ground, we would nail, to the pole, a "one by four" board about six or seven feet long. This board would parallel the ground. Another board of similar size would be nailed at a right angle just above the first board.

Using pitchforks, the dried plants with the peanuts would then be stacked around the pole with those two boards keeping them off the ground. This way they would not soak up moisture from the ground. In a few weeks, the peanuts would have dried. Someone with a "peanut picker" would come to our farm. Dried plants with the peanuts would be fed into the picker. It would separate the peanuts from the plants, with the peanuts going into a bag. The plants would come out separately in "hay bales," to be used for cow feed. Later, the process was more mechanized. The "stacks" were eliminated and the plants were left on the ground to dry. Rain could slow the process.

When the peanuts were dry, a machine would come along picking the plants off the ground and separating the peanuts from the plants, which were still baled. The bales were hauled to the barn and stored out of the weather and used later to feed the livestock. The peanuts were taken to the peanut mill for processing. Daddy's mom, my grandmother, worked there for years, until she retired when I was still in grammar school.

After peanuts, it was time to start picking cotton. While I was at home, we were still picking it by hand. A bag about six feet long would be pulled with a strap that went over a shoulder. I would go down a row of cotton picking it and putting it in the bag. It was "back breaking" work, up and down and side to side. My back would get so tired and sore that I would often crawl on my knees to get some momentary relief for my back. Mom would make "pads" for our knees to protect them from the hot dirt and sandspurs. Temperatures were often in the nineties. The dirt would be so hot my feet would burn.

When the bag was full with thirty or forty pounds of cotton it was emptied into a truck nearby. Each bag was weighed and a tally kept of how much each person picked. When the truck was full it was taken to the gin about ten miles away. The gin would separate the cotton from the seeds. The cotton would be bundled in bales and sent to the cotton mills to make thread and cloth. This was used for many purposes, including making clothes. The seed was used for making meal for feed for the livestock, or cotton seed oil for multiple purposes, or used to plant the next crop.

School started in late August or early September. I was glad to have a break from the drudgery of the farm and to see my friends.

Quite often, cotton would still be in the fields. We would come home from school and pick cotton until it was all harvested. One year, a hurricane was coming and we still had cotton in the field. That was the second time that I missed a half day of school to work. Daddy came to pick us up from school and we picked cotton the rest of the day. Sure enough, the rains came. When rain knocked cotton to the ground it would be harder to harvest, damaged to some extent, and bring a lower price at the gin. We would be finished with cotton sometime in September and, by then, it was time to start gathering corn.

For some people, this was a cash crop, like cotton, peanuts, and watermelons were for us. We grew it primarily as food for us and the livestock.

While it was young and starting to mature, we would eat the corn. Sometimes it was eaten on the cob. Sometimes it was cut from the cob and canned in jars. In later years, it would be stored in a freezer. Throughout the year, matured dry corn was taken to the mill and ground into cornmeal. We had cornbread all year long, sometimes fried and sometimes baked.

When the corn had fully matured by the fall, the kernels hardened and the husks turned brown. The hard work followed. In the early years, we did it all by hand. We called it "pulling corn." To me, this was one of the most miserable jobs on the farm.

By September, the hottest temperatures of 90 and 100 degrees had passed, but it was still hot much of the time.

When the corn was small, the rows were clean, plowed frequently enough to eliminate the weeds. As the stalks of corn grew higher, the plowing stopped. By the time the corn was grown the weeds were sometimes just as tall as the corn.

When we "pulled corn" we used the same bag we had previously used for cotton. We would break off the corn, ear by ear, and put it in the bag. This was some of the work I hated most.

Bruce Pelham

The temperatures were still hot and in between those rows of corn we couldn't feel a breeze. The husk would stick to the body. It wouldn't take long before my body would be stinging. This would last all day. Periodically, we would empty the 30 to 40 pound bags into a trailer, to be taken to the barn later. In the barn the corn was stored in a large room called the corncrib. It was fed to the livestock all through the year. Each year before we started gathering corn, we would have to clean out the crib. Keep in mind that this crib was used to store corn, primarily to feed livestock.

We would spend all day removing old tassels, cornhusks, dirt and dust from the crib. We swept until it was as clean as the house in which we lived, or so we thought. The next morning, my father would take us out to the barn to inspect our work from the day before. After walking around and looking at the corncrib he would take his hand and rub his fingers across the top of the window frame. It would have some dust, of course. He would look at it, frowning, and say, "It's still dirty, do it again. And this time, do it right." That would be our job for another day. We would take buckets of soapy water and scrub the place. The next day the same thing would happen. It was never good enough. There was always room for improvement. That was the message. That was always the message. "As long as there was room for improvement, we should be working to do it right." Not a bad message, only Daddy's criticism rarely was accompanied by, or followed with, compliments or encouragement.

Baling hay took place in spring or summer, in between crops. Very few people owned hay baling equipment. Someone who did would come through baling and we would pay him so much per bale.

Very often, weather would have a huge impact on the hay crops. When the hay was cut, it was still filled with moisture. If it was baled with moisture still in the grass, it would get hot inside and rot.

If we were fortunate enough for it to dry and be baled before the rain, we loaded it onto a wagon, or trailer, to be transported to the barn. This was a hot stinging job. If stacked in the barn wet, it would spoil. Today, you will see giant rolls of hay that stay in the fields until eaten by the livestock.

The loft of the barn was used to store the hay, which fed the livestock through the winter, when very little was growing. If we didn't have enough, we had to buy more hay or start selling cows early, usually at less favorable prices.

I didn't like loading and unloading hay. The bales weighed 30-40 pounds and lifting them was exhausting work. It was a hot job, even in the fall, just like pulling corn. Particles of the corn tassels or hay would be all over us and it would sting like crazy. Much of the day would be spent like that. You could wash it off at lunchtime and as soon as you returned to work, it was back again and the stinging renewed.

In spite of the work, summer was the most peaceful time of the year in many ways. Daddy was truly a man "possessed." By his own demons. When we were all consumed with work, he wasn't so concerned about what we were doing. His philosophy of keeping us busy produced a family of workaholics like he was.

I still remember the day in 1963, when I had told him I was leaving home. Throughout the last couple of months of my senior year of high school, he kept reminding me to get my application in to Chipola Junior College. I finally said, "I'm not going to Chipola, I'm going to FSU." For a long moment, I thought he was going to hit me. He finally said, "If you do that, don't expect a penny from me." I said, "I don't." I could feel his tension. Finally, he said, "If you will help me gather the crops, I will take you to Tallahassee in time for school." My brother Stan intended to farm. He bought 40 acres across the road from my Dad when he got out of the Air Force. He very quickly decided farming was not what he wanted to do. I don't think Dad ever contemplated that we would all choose to leave that life behind.

I worked all summer and he took me and my older brother, Jerry, to Tallahassee. Having finished Chipola, Jerry was starting his junior year at FSU. He had excelled at Chipola in spite of the long hours he had spent in the fields every day when he got home. Mom worked hard in helping us to secure housing scholarships at

FSU collecting many letters of recommendation that were required for our applications.

I started to college at Florida State University in 1963. I sometimes worked forty to fifty hours per week while going to school and taking a full academic load. These were also particularly turbulent times. The county where I grew up had been totally segregated when I was in school. That changed during my first year at FSU.

I got a close up look at picketing and sit-down demonstrations at the local restaurants, especially the ones near campus. One vivid memory has haunted me for decades. On my way home from class, I had to walk past a popular campus-side restaurant. One day a large crowd had gathered to watch as students picketed in protest of the segregated status of the restaurant. As we stood there watching, a car drove slowly by. One of its occupants threw an egg filled with something that badly burned the face of the picketer that it hit.

Black high school students boycotted their schools in protest of segregation and discrimination in funding of their schools. Those kids attended class in churches on those days. I cut my own classes and worked as a teacher in one of those churches during the boycotts.

The doors of the church I was attending during my freshman year were locked because a group of African students had the audacity to walk up the steps to the church on "International Students Day." I got to vote in the election when that three-thousand-member church voted to remain segregated. Almost half of the membership voted to integrate the church, as slightly over half voted to keep it segregated. I was sick. As I left the church that night, the black janitor had already started to sweep the floors in the balcony. I found another church. Those were stressful times for all of us.

One of the most horrifying events of my life happened in November of 1963, during my freshman year at FSU. President John F. Kennedy was assassinated. The whole world was crazy. I was severely depressed for some time and very uneasy about what was happening. When I was in college, Dad was active in the Klan. This was in the mid-sixties.

In 1964, during the Presidential election, my youngest brother Richard, five years younger than me, wrote a letter to the editor of the nearest daily newspaper in support of Lyndon Johnson over Barry Goldwater in the presidential election. My father was enraged.

What bothered him, of course, was that some of his fellow Klansmen would hold him responsible for his son's political views. "What would the neighbors think?"

He ordered Richard to write a letter to the editor retracting his "misguided" support of Johnson. Richard had gone through several revisions of the letter and none were satisfactory to my father. This is an example of the hypocrisy often exhibited by him. We were always supposed to tell the truth yet he forced my brother to lie. We were always told to treat everybody as equals only this did not apply to African Americans. They weren't "people" to him. Richard did, under threat of physical harm, write the letter saying he was misinformed.

Richard called me and explained what was happening. I rented a car and drove home, hoping to be able to reason with my father. I should have known better. He would not agree for Richard to retract the second letter. I called the editor and explained the situation but he would not agree to pull the retraction letter. He agreed to print a letter from me immediately following Richard's retraction letter in the same edition. My letter explained that Richard had been forced to write that letter by our father. I told Dad what would be in the paper. He was furious. He came out of his easy chair in the living room. The "haymaker" he threw would have flattened me if he had connected. I knew better than to react. His fist stopped only inches from my face.

In 1968, more insanity followed. Martin Luther King, Jr. was assassinated as he battled for racial equality. Robert Kennedy was shot and killed in his own bid for the Presidency. To make it even more horrifying, all of this was televised live for the whole world to see. The United States, the world leader of Democracy, was embroiled in "Third World anarchy."

I started law school in 1968, having worked for a year after graduation from college.

The turbulence continued. The Viet Nam War had been going on for some time. The FSU campus was again a hot bed of student activism. Students had taken over administration buildings at universities all over the country in protest of the war.

The local sheriff had the FSU administration building surrounded by uniformed National Guardsmen with drawn bayonets to prevent that from happening at FSU. Unbelievable! At Kent State University, the National Guard fired upon demonstrating college students, killing some of them. Those days were sometimes exciting; sometimes depressing; sometimes scary; and always really stressful.

About half way through law school, I joined the National Guard, later transferring to the Army Reserve, and avoided going to Viet Nam. There no longer were deferments for being in school; for being married; or, for having children. I was married with a newborn baby and in basic training at twenty-five. Seven years off the farm and in the classroom had left me in terrible physical condition. I was there with eighteen and nineteen year olds.

That period of my life was chaotic and stressful. Earlier I tried to enlist and wasn't accepted for medical reasons. That was before I had concluded that this war was a travesty.

Those of you who have been through that basic military training know how stressful it is. Those of you who haven't probably would not understand no matter how good I was at explaining it. Just like those of us who did not go to Viet Nam, could not possibly understand what it was like to be there. That kind of stress has to be experienced to understand it. Our involvement in wars in the Middle East has gone on for over a decade. How many hundreds of years had these wars gone on before we got involved? The stress for the participants has to be horrific. My life has involved lots of stress and I would not begin to equate it with the kind of stress those fighting soldiers endure.

I returned from basic training to finish law school. While in law school I got involved in the real estate business. For years I was involved in sales, developing, building, and finance. All of this was highly stressful. I took a beating ... mentally, financially, and emotionally. I was divorced twice and know that I was responsible for my divorces which were, for me, more stressful than anything I could experience other than the loss of loved ones. Many years after all of this my multiple sclerosis symptoms started surfacing.

This chapter is about my "growing up." It has taken many twists and turns. My learning experiences were filled with much difficulty. I am still growing. I have learned a lot about multiple sclerosis and its effect on my body in the process. I decided to share my journey with you; especially my recovery. It wasn't easy and it has been a real learning experience. I encourage YOU to take charge of YOUR healthcare and your life. You probably have more power than you realize.

Our bodies were created to function properly. We do much to interfere with this. Stress contributes to many diseases, including MS.

I take responsibility for all of the opinions and judgments in this chapter. Some of you may agree with them. Some may strongly disagree. I ask you to understand that I am writing about things that affected my life. I ask you to consider your own history and what effect your life may have had on your own journey, including your experience with MS.

In the following chapters I look at stress, a likely "trigger" of MS, what I did to reduce it in my life and the likely effect it had on my recovery from this horrible disease.

All healing is essentially the release from fear.
-- A Course in Miracles

It takes a lot of courage to release the familiar ... in change there is power. *– Alan Cohen*

Chapter 5

The Rock Slide
(Stress and Its Effects)

Use the pain in your life to create something meaningful.
-- Bernie S. Siegel, M.D.

Stress is difficult to define and people don't necessarily mean the same thing when they talk about it. It appears that multiple sclerosis brings its own kind of stress.

If this is true, then stress is included in the cause and the effect. I stress over "being stressed" which makes my condition worse.

Some people with MS are offended by the suggestion that they play a part, any part, in the causation of the disease. They are much more content to think in terms of the disease happening to them. For me, it was encouraging to know that maybe I could "undo" or correct some of the damage that I had done.

The truth is that reality begins in the mind. Whatever I do begins, on some level, in the mind. For example, I move into the oncoming lane in order to pass the car in front of me. I run head on into a tractor-trailer. This started in the mind with "I am going to pass that car in front of me." Why someone would do that, I don't know. The conscious mind doesn't always know. What I do know is that I put myself in a position to be hit by that truck. I "decided to change lanes."

Just because I don't understand the part I play in creating a disease in my body, doesn't mean that "it just happened to me." Just because research has not definitively proven a causal relationship between stress and multiple sclerosis doesn't mean that it doesn't exist. Just because we cannot prove the existence of mankind prior to this one here on earth, doesn't mean that mankind never existed before.

Many attempts have been made to show a connection between stress and exacerbations of multiple sclerosis. Studies have been conducted and published on this possible connection. One such study was published in a British medical journal.

This study definitely indicates a connection between the two, but certainly is not conclusive. Several studies also address other factors such as medications, geography, viral or bacterial infections, and time. There are problems in establishing conclusive links with the various factors.

Some studies have indicated that stress is more important than was previously known. According to them, stress doesn't just come and go, but goes to our very core. And it alters our bodies including our brain. Our bodies become sensitized to stress. Then, it takes very little to trigger that response. Chemicals are released into the body causing the body to react. The body basically "rewires itself as a protection." Experiencing everyday occurrences may then trigger an inappropriate reaction.

Research has shown that people become sensitized to stress and this actually alters physical patterns in the brain. Then the body just reacts to the stress. Some theorize that a serious event, like losing a parent when the child is young, is harder to overcome than when older. This may, in fact, permanently "rewire" the brain, leaving it less able to handle everyday stress.

This would indicate a link between some psychological event and some later physical reaction. I am sure this was true with my father. The events of his childhood triggered extreme reactions in him as an adult. Unstable home life, abusive parents, alcoholics, and other extended crises could have a profound effect on a person for many years to come, possibly for their entire lives. Today, I think very few people would question the connection between psychological stress and physical factors such as fatigue or headaches.

There seems to be a connection between how we handle stress today and what kind of stress we may have previously suffered. It seems to have an effect on those areas of the brain controlling such basics as eating and immune responses, or lack of them. Studies have shown the same basic reactions involving such different events as extreme exercise, the death of someone close, or pressure at work. Some have theorized that a stress response system in previous generations was needed to protect us from life threatening situations rather than our everyday frustrations and disappointments.

What we call the stress system is responsible for much more than just our response to stress. Hormones generated affect the immune system, the cardiovascular system, and so much else. Short term memory is affected. Communication between brain cells is directly affected. Stress alters serotonin pathways and is linked with depression. Most likely, the chemicals being released in response to stress are triggering physical reactions throughout the body. Damage is made to blood cells; heart attacks and strokes are caused; the immune system is damaged. Stress hormones are thought to be connected to rheumatoid arthritis. Studies have shown a strong link with strokes, even many years after the event occurred. Many chemicals are released and the effects are far reaching.

There has long been evidence that psychological stress actually changes the brain's makeup. Just picture what extended torture can do to a person. And when the trauma happens to a child, it may not even occur to us to connect that trauma to him having a heart attack or some other disease years later. Very often, the way a person handles a current event may have much to do with what had happened in his earlier life. Likewise, it may have a great deal to do with his health later in his life.

In studying the disease and any correlation to specific factors involves going back in time. Memory is far from totally accurate. Small details may be eliminated completely. Large details may end up being related in a way that was totally unrealistic if viewed precisely when it happened.

With myself, for example, I have had the opportunity to explore lots of memory failure as it pertains to me specifically. I have my memory, or recall, of particular events in my life. Then, I have the memories of people, family members or friends, who were a part of those memories. Their recall may not, necessarily, agree with mine. This doesn't mean that one is "right" and the other is "wrong." It may just mean that the memories, and not the facts, are different. It may be, even at the time, that what I experienced is not what they experienced. Much study has been done on this phenomenon in a totally different arena.

Criminologists have long recognized that two witnesses of the same event will remember it differently. In fact, they saw it differently. Each can sit on the witness stand and truthfully testify, under oath, to having seen the same event happen in two totally distinct ways.

People have sat in prisons, and do today, for decades that were innocent. Certainly, some of this was intentional. Just as certainly, in other cases the witnesses have been convinced of their own testimony, only to have it disproven years later, by DNA evidence. What was witnessed, for whatever reason, was simply different.

It is the same as trying to determine what particular event played what part in the health of any single person. I have all of the records from visits with my neurologist, covering eighteen years. I have read his observations concerning my disease at various times during that period. His notes from each visit contain observations he makes, reports that I give to him, and his own personal conclusion based on those events. Notes I made after those visits do not always concur with his observations of those visits. I have very clear memories of certain events that took place that are not reflected in his notes. Obviously some things that were memorable to me did not seem that important to him.

What I don't have is an accurate chronology of my entire life. The causative events possibly would be found there, rather than in studying the symptoms which are noticeable today. I have looked, and am still looking, at the possible causative factors contained in my background.

This depends, in large part, on the accuracy of my memory. I have acknowledged the reasons why this is not necessarily accurate. My recollections are colored by what was going on with me at the time and by everything that has happened to me since.

I don't believe that stress, alone, causes multiple sclerosis. I believe that a propensity to have the disease exists in some people and I believe that some other factor, or factors, such as stress, will trigger responses in the body which we know as multiple sclerosis.

Stress, like so many other things, is not all bad. One purpose, actually, is to protect you. It does this by causing chemicals to be released in the body with results that are sometimes simply amazing.

Consequently, reaction times sharply increase and the mind moves at much greater speed. Most of us have heard stories of seemingly super human feats. For example, a man comes upon an accident with a car overturned and a man trapped underneath. Without hesitation, he rushes to the car and picks up one corner, enabling the man to be pulled free. Ordinarily, that man could not do this. But he did it during an extremely stressful event.

The main hormone released during stress is cortisol. A derivative, prednisone, is sometimes used to treat multiple sclerosis. It has been suggested by some that stress may not cause the problem but, instead, may itself be caused by the drop in levels of cortisol.

I will point out here that having more than one autoimmune disease is not uncommon. This may present some challenging treatment problems.

I have several, which I will discuss at a later time. But this one presents a good, typical example. While prednisone may very well be effective in treating MS, it may also send blood sugar levels through the roof. To rather frightening levels, I might add. Prednisone, in my case, triggered pancreatitis which was incredibly painful and can be deadly.

Another interesting possibility presents itself. Rather than stress causing the exacerbations, maybe this happens in reverse order. Maybe the exacerbations come first and then the stress. If it happens that you feel stressed at a time when no exacerbation is developing, then nothing happens. The suggestion is that stress by itself may not be enough to cause an exacerbation.

Whichever one comes first most everyone acknowledges the importance of managing stress. Withdrawing from stressful situations may result in other stresses. Quitting a stressful job and staying home, for example, just produces new stresses. Some stresses such as depression may come from within, but be affected by outward events such as noise. With most things, no two people are affected exactly the same way, or to the same extent. Medicines affect people differently. What works for me may not work in the same way for you. The same is true of foods. What raises your blood sugar may not have the same effect on mine.

In one well-documented case a patient resorted to hypnosis out of desperation. She had suffered severe pain caused by her multiple sclerosis-related nerve damage. Nothing else had worked for her. It took only a couple of sessions. She wanted to help other people and she began the study of hypnosis. As she noted, hypnosis doesn't eliminate the stress, but does cause a person to respond differently. Chronic pain is really debilitating. Relieving the stress of feeling uncomfortable and never getting proper rest is very therapeutic. Dr. Kerry Abaco, a doctor of Oriental Medicine, has treated me successfully for pain with acupuncture on more than one occasion. This has been so successful with me that I really have to question the motives of doctors who simply prescribe pills for pain rather than send the patient out for acupuncture treatments.

People turn to different things including acupuncture, exercise, meditation, prayer groups, or psychotherapy to help with pain and other stressful situations. Stress is a normal part of life, and everyone goes through it differently.

As previously stated, the relationship between MS and stress is certainly not a proven fact. There is no question that stress contributes to the elevation of my blood sugar. I am convinced that it was a contributing factor to my MS and other illnesses as well. The stress of other illnesses on my body, like the flu, has that same effect. It has long been accepted that stress may be a contributing factor with some heart problems.

As previously noted, life itself includes a certain amount of stress for most everyone. From college all the way through my adult life, choices I made contributed directly to my heightened stress. Multiple sclerosis adds its own particular stressful occurrences including the completely unpredictable course of the disease. The effects of stress may be different for each of us, like upsetting or knotting our stomachs, or greatly increasing our perspiration. Many people with MS experience more symptoms during stressful times. Removal of the stress seems to reduce the symptoms or, at least, their severity. Therefore, learning to relax may be a critical element of learning to live with the disease. It is important to understand as much as possible about stress and the part it plays in multiple sclerosis. Relaxing doesn't just happen. Quite often it takes a very special effort and a great deal of motivation and practice.

The emotional challenges of MS are almost too numerous to discuss here. Many people suffer bouts of severe depression. Others become very irritable and great mood swings are not uncommon.

It is very important to simplify one's daily life. Complications seem to increase stress and effects of MS in general. Learning muscle relaxation techniques can be essential to those who suffer muscle cramps and even severe pain. Deep breathing exercises and visualization techniques have benefitted many. Managing anger becomes an integral part of a successful therapeutic process. Learning to dissipate anger or channel it into a positive force may be very beneficial.

While these things may go a long way toward assisting the mind to deal with multiple sclerosis, there are also different things that will assist the body in battling its own decline.

Many years ago the Oriental art of self-defense, Tai Chi, was very instrumental in assisting me on the road to recovery. I still remember when I first spoke with the head of the Tai Chi center in Tallahassee. I explained to him the problems that I had with memory, or recall, and the problems I could envision with trying to remember all the different moves.

He was great. He suggested that we start with one move and increase it, one by one, until we reached four moves. That was not too many for me to recall. I practiced those in several sessions, until I felt comfortable with them. Then he added another. And then another. Until eventually, I was going through the entire sequence.

There is absolutely no question in my mind that my balance and strength improved tremendously. I didn't do it long enough to become proficient at it, but I made great strides in balance, coordination, strength, and recall. I discontinued it because I had the opportunity to go back to work full-time. There simply wasn't time for everything I wanted to do.

Again, I don't think we ever reach the point where it would not be helpful and healthful. Deep breathing and slow, gentle movements are the primary elements of this exercise, sometimes referred to as moving meditation. For those whose MS has progressed too far to allow participation in normal Tai Chi, a modified version can be done sitting down.

Exercise, in general, may help and comes in many forms that may assist in living with multiple sclerosis. It doesn't matter if it is swimming, working out in a gym or at home, playing golf or just plain walking. Exercise is beneficial, period. Massage and body work is often used to relax muscles, reduce stress and relieve other conditions made worse by muscle tension.

Yoga can be a very therapeutic exercise for people with MS. It emphasizes relaxation, breathing and deliberate movements, all of which can be great therapies for relieving stress and for multiple sclerosis.

Relaxation is a state of deep rest that can change the effects of stressful thoughts. This may be accomplished by repeating a prayer, word, sound, phrase, or some muscular activity.

In the next chapter we explore the effect that all of this has on the decline of cognition. As is the case with many people, the greatest stress in my life came in the earliest years of my life. How much it affected the course of my disease no one knows. For me, I am certain that it had some effect on my eventual experience with MS and on my loss of cognition.

The greatest gift you can give yourself is joy ... it will produce wonders in your life.
-- Jack Boland

Be grateful for whatever comes because each has been sent as a guide from beyond.   *-- Rumi*

Chapter 6

Weathering the Storm
(Decline of Cognition)

Learn to accept the spiritual flat tires in life that redirect you to the creator's schedule.   -- Bernie S. Siegel, M.D.

Cognition means "to know." It involves what we think of as the functions of the brain. It may involve any, or all, of our senses of sight, hearing, taste, touch and smell.

Knowledge is comprised of memories involving the functions of knowing, remembering, and processing all of this information.

Cognition assists us in reaching our goals. Our past and our memories point us in the right direction. Something as simple as taking a long walk involves this process. What destination do I want to reach? How much time do I have? What route do I take? How fast will I have to walk?

The act of taking a walk will involve all of these decisions, and more. What is amazing is how little time it takes for all of this process to take place. I can think of walking, destination, route, time, etc., in little more than an instant.

The easiest way to understand what cognition means is to substitute the word "thinking." It covers a broad spectrum of activities. The seemingly simple task of paying attention is included in this list. It covers learning and remembering all kinds of information. I am reminded of that period of time when I was learning to spell colors and associate the pictures of those colors with the words; of slowly reciting the first few numbers; and learning to say my "a-b-c's." Learning these basics was challenging at the time. Adding and subtracting numbers became easier and by the time I started learning my multiplication tables, it was fun for me. Using language to communicate was something that was easier as I matured. Many years later, in real estate, I could figure the monthly amount of an amortized mortgage payment in my head and be very close to the actual amount.

Cognitive abnormalities in multiple sclerosis patients may affect some or all of those activities. Initially, these may be minor and very subtle, growing into major disabilities as the disease progresses. Deficiency in the areas of short term memory and thought processing creates great difficulty in the functions of concentrating and reasoning, which once seemed so natural to me.

Growing up in a three bedroom house with my parents and four siblings taught me to improvise. I studied with the radio playing all the way through high school. My parents were constantly asking, "How can you study with all of that noise?" The truth is, "that noise" (white noise) enabled me to concentrate. It blocked out all of the real noise, and I could study quite effectively. I continued that through college. I would go sit in the student union or some student-filled restaurant near campus and study for hours. In the library, I would be distracted by the sound of a pencil dropping or someone coughing.

For me, cognition was always one of my strengths. I was aware of this in high school. I became more aware of it as the years passed and I recognized it for what it was.

In 2010, writing this book, I noticed that my cognitive ability had declined over the years. I might have thought it was a recent occurrence except that months before I had come across some notes I made which were dated five years before. At least that far back I had noticed that my cognitive ability didn't seem to be as good as it once was.

During the last year, I have spent lots of time writing. There have been more times for me to notice when my cognition was not functioning well. It would sometimes interfere with things I was trying to do. If I had been doing something less strenuous mentally, I may not have noticed. The same may be true if I had not been growing older and reached the point that I was aware of the declining mental abilities of some older people.

When visiting an assisted living facility, I was reminded that some people maintain their mental abilities well. And I couldn't help but notice, when visiting there, that everyone in that facility was not mentally alert. Many are less and less active. Some have lost interest, "given up." Some residents are just existing. At the same time, some are incredibly alert.

My mom has been a real role model for me with her dedication to walking. The same is true as I watch her with games. Some are on TV and some are in books. They serve to maintain that mental sharpness she always had.

Experiences and trends give us an idea of what the future might hold. To make sense of the near infinite details of our surroundings, a large part of cognition involves the organization of our thoughts. These cognitive categories are not always really distinct. Perception, attention and memory are necessary to organize the processes involved in how we think.

Perception might let you know that you're hungry. Memory plays a really important part in this process and it might be short term memory, or long term memory, or subconscious memory. Memory might give you some idea of what you want to eat to satisfy this hunger. Another function enables you to do all the planning required for satisfying your hunger. It might involve thinking about cooking and where the different items are that you need for your meal. It might involve you picking up the telephone to order take-out or delivery.

Cognitive impairment is when there is a problem with perceiving, thinking or remembering. This could be caused by head injuries, by a stroke, or some chronic disease such as multiple sclerosis. Symptoms could relate to short term memory or to problem solving, or to both. It may just relate to attention span. It might entail having a problem finding the right word to use in a conversation.

Cognitive dysfunction as a symptom of multiple sclerosis affects patients in different ways. It is one that has caused me the most noticeable, lasting problems. Not noticeable in the sense that everyone can see them, but noticeable in the sense that they caused me functional difficulties. It also is the kind of symptom that is not so easily understood as, for example, difficulty in walking. This, everybody can see and relate to. It may be similar to the kind of problem that some people notice when they get older, or when involved in an activity such as having responsibility for kids.

A significant problem with my memory has had to do with short term deficiencies. I notice it at times when I am in the middle of a sentence and all of a sudden my mind goes blank and I can't remember what I had been talking about. Or, when a word won't come to me. It is very noticeable when I pick up the phone to call someone and lose all recollection of who it was I was about to call, or why. At times I have gone to the grocery store to get some specific item and then, as I get my buggy to push down the aisle, my mind goes blank. I have no idea what it is that brought me to the grocery store.

For years now I have used a pill box for my medicine. Sometimes, I could not remember when I had taken it last. Even now, after years of sorting my medications in a pill box for a week at a time, I sometimes have to go look at my pill box in order to know if I have taken my medicine. Very often I realize that I have taken the medicine because that compartment is empty, and I will have no memory of having taken it. It is just something I learned to live with. In taking my insulin for my diabetes three times daily, I have to keep a little notebook next to my insulin. I note when I take it or I end up in that same situation of having taken it already and having no memory of doing so.

When it came to performing abstract tasks, I would have to be very, very careful not to lose track of what I was doing. This was important in practicing law. For three years I did not work. For four more years I worked in a non-legal position. By then, I was very conscious of what could happen and I learned to work around it.

One thing I would do is limit the number of cases I was working on at any one time. I learned to keep very detailed notes in each file as to exactly where I was in the process of completing that case. Without those notes, it would have been easy to forget exactly where I was with that file.

I spent many years of my life having a very efficient memory, one that sometimes reminded me of a small computer. It stored and organized so much knowledge that it often was not necessary for me to keep detailed notes because I would know exactly what I was supposed to be doing with each task, all of the time.

Later, when I tried to work on too many cases at one time they would start to overlap. The stress would cause everything to run together and me to feel confused about where I was on each file. I mastered this simply by staying very organized, with the help of great assistants, and being very sequential in my daily practice. It simply would not have worked for me to keep too many active files going at the same time.

For most of my life, I was always able to work on several different things at the same time, or multi-task. With MS, it is much more difficult to keep my mind on several different things at one time.

For me, and for lots of people with multiple sclerosis, the mind simply cannot take in as much information as it once did and keep it properly prioritized. I have noticed that it takes me more time to process information, to hear someone speaking and know instantly what they're talking about.

Problems with cognition actually are very common among people who have MS. Estimates vary, but somewhere between one-third and two-thirds of people with multiple sclerosis suffer problems with cognition to some extent. Sometimes it is so subtle that the person doesn't even notice it, or doesn't attribute it to MS. And, it doesn't follow the same path with everyone. It isn't that with multiple sclerosis you suffer cognitive impairment and it gets worse and worse as time goes by. It may be that you have some problem with cognition and it stays relatively constant over a long period of time. It may be that you have a problem with cognition and it grows slowly worse, as other symptoms of MS grow slowly worse.

Problems with cognition seem to follow along with more permanent destruction of brain tissue. With my own cognitive problems, I'm sure it was happening long before I noticed it. This symptom was a more permanent one than other symptoms I had with multiple sclerosis. As my symptoms in general have improved over the years, I discovered that my cognitive function did not exactly return to where it was. Certain damage was done to the nervous system which was permanent. I had continued to notice over a period of years that I had this dysfunction. Because of my writing, I noticed it more than I ever had before. I discussed it with my doctor and he arranged for me to be tested in a very comprehensive way.

The testing lasted two hours and then was reviewed at length by a team of professionals. They confirmed what I suspected. My cognitive abilities had suffered. The truth is that damage creating the dysfunction had occurred many years ago. My other symptoms improved, but this one did not because the damage was permanent.

A very common symptom of MS, as with many other diseases, is depression. In that case, cognitive function seems to be affected including memory, attention, and ability to concentrate. People who are depressed often have trouble making good decisions, especially quick or complicated decisions like the ones that confront us in everyday life.

The most common symptom of multiple sclerosis is fatigue and is experienced by probably eighty to ninety percent of people with MS. It also is considered one of the most debilitating symptoms, leaving one less able to perform everyday life functions. The fatigue felt by people with MS may very well affect the way they perform cognitively. Intolerance of heat, in people with multiple sclerosis, can make most all symptoms of MS worse. And this applies to cognitive dysfunction.

In summary, while cognitive dysfunction may not outwardly be the most common symptom of multiple sclerosis, it certainly has been one of the most debilitating for me. Even when I had trouble walking or talking, the cognitive dysfunction was still the one that caused me the most problems. I lived most of my life under more than normal stress. In my opinion, prolonged stress takes its toll on cognition which was discussed in Chapter 5.

See your day as a classroom … life is a great teacher.
— Bernie S. Siegel, M.D.

Ask and it will be given to you …
-- Matthew 7:7

Step up to the microphone and repeat your question so it gets heard and recorded on God's answering machine. How God answers and who God uses to answer may surprise you.
— Bernie S. Siegel, M.D.

Chapter 7

Starting the Climb

(Unity, Prayer and Attitude)

It is your attitude at the beginning of a difficult task which, more than anything else, will affect its successful outcome.

-- William James

The first time I went to a Unity church was in 1993. I remember like it was yesterday. I had recently started seeing my neurologist because of strange symptoms that had been going on with me. Already, I had slowed the pace of my life. My daughter, Lori, had asked me more than once to go to church with her and a friend. I never had. Now, I wasn't quite so "busy."

Spiritual and physical mishaps sometimes have a way of redirecting our schedules.

We went to church on the first night of a twelve week workshop. I had no idea then what an enlightening and life altering experience it was to be. The church was originally a residence that had been converted to a church many years before. When I walked into that church the first time, I felt very peaceful, and at home.

Participants in this workshop were asked to make several commitments as a prerequisite for attending the workshop. One was to attend church, there, all twelve weeks. Another was to volunteer for, and perform, some job at the church for the duration of the twelve week period. I told Lori that I would like to do some job that involved working with teenagers. She checked with the minister's assistant, a young woman named Robin, about my request.

I loved her response and her sense of humor. Upon learning that I would like to work with teenagers, she asked, "Is he nuts, or what?" And she smiled, with so much understanding. Then she said, "Have him go over and talk to Kathy, who is the YOU (Youth of Unity) sponsor, and volunteer to assist her." I did that the following Sunday and of course she welcomed me. I finished the twelve week workshop and I worked with Kathy as a YOU sponsor for the next three years. Then, and for many years since, she has been such an inspiration to me. She is truly a miracle and an angel for so many people.

The group did a lot of traveling, usually to retreats for a weekend. One of my jobs as a sponsor was to travel with the teenagers as a chaperone. I travelled with them to different camps in Florida and once, with four of them for a week to Unity Village, Missouri, the home of Unity School of Christianity.

For them and for me these trips were truly inspirational. I was in the early stages of my MS and balance problems were already very noticeable. On one trip, the campers were engaged in several challenging activities that involved lots of discipline and teamwork. As a sponsor I was expected to participate. Keenly aware of my growing physical limitations, I would have chosen, on my own, not to participate in some of the activities. With them, this was not an option.

A large log lay on the ground. The task was to walk the log without falling off. When they walked on the log, so did I. One of them would be in front of me, for me to touch and maintain my balance. Another would be behind me, also assisting me in staying balanced. There was more doubt in me than there was in all of them. They expected me to participate and assisted me in doing it successfully. I felt more surprise than I saw on any of their faces.

Fifteen feet up in the air, a rope was strung tightly from one tree to another. A little higher than waist-level were two more ropes to hold onto as I walked the tightrope. Those who have done "a ropes course" will recognize some of the activities. One of them placed himself right in front of me as I walked and one was right behind me, ready to lend assistance if it was needed. I made it all of the way across with no major mishaps. It was nothing short of invigorating.

When it came time to do the "backward fall," I didn't even hesitate. I was no longer apprehensive. A part of what the ropes course was designed for had been accomplished. I trusted them and they trusted me. More importantly, I trusted myself. I was standing on a platform probably 12-15 feet in the air. I walked to the edge and then I turned my back to the open side.

Below was a group of teenagers, ages 13-17, peering up at me. They made two parallel lines facing each other. Each line extended both hands toward the other one, an arm's length apart. When someone said, "Go," I fell backward. My feet remained in place as my head arched downward, off the platform. My feet left the platform as my head reached their level. Then I was falling straight down, horizontally, totally trusting that group of young people to protect me from hitting the ground.

They caught me, of course. I cannot even begin to explain how empowering that whole experience was. By then, I knew they would catch me. That wasn't the surprise. The surprise was that they seemed to do it so effortlessly, without dropping me. I landed, on those hands, in a totally horizontal position, as I expected. What I didn't expect was to see them hardly move as they caught me. It was as if I had rolled off my bed and landed on a pair of mattresses lying on the floor, adjacent to my bed.

Those are just some examples of the empowering experiences I had with those young people in the early days of my journey with multiple sclerosis. I was reminded of one of the many gems left to us by Mark Twain ... "To succeed in life, you need two things – ignorance and confidence." Our attitudes have such an impact on what goes on in our lives.

The greatest discovery of my generation is that human beings, by changing the inner attitudes of their minds, can change the outer aspects of their lives.
-- William James

At that same church, we had a visiting minister one day who was going to be conducting a "fire walking" workshop the following week, I had heard of this seemingly foolish game before. Lori asked me if I was interested in participating. I said sure and we did. I will explain the whole process, not so as to bore you, but to demonstrate a point this book is intended to convey. Every ACTION starts in the mind, as a thought. We can say "yes" to life.

We started the process that evening, stacking logs in a vertical fashion, making a large teepee-like structure that was probably twelve feet high. The bottom of the teepee was packed with very flammable brush. All of it was covered with a lighter fluid to make it burn evenly and quickly. The fire was ignited with the simple toss of a match, followed by a huge, instant bonfire. After the fire was ablaze, we all went inside a nearby building for our very detailed instructions. This lasted over an hour while the fire outside blazed.

One of the ladies assisting with the instruction had some experience with fire walking, not all good. She had once burned the soles of her feet very badly, having not paid close attention to the instructions. I trusted the instructors, including her, and listened attentively. They had my full attention with every word they spoke. One of the most important messages was to "be present." I frequently have to remind myself that today is all we have and to live it accordingly.

When we returned to our giant bonfire, it had been reduced to a huge pile of brightly burning coals. We took rakes and spread the coals, making a large rectangle. It was probably twenty feet long and almost as wide. The ground was completely covered with burning coals so hot that they were white with bits of red peeking through.

The instructions were to walk quickly and steadily across that bed of coals, with bare feet. Someone said the temperature inside the mountain of coals had been several hundred degrees. The intensity was much less when the coals were spread. Still hot enough, however, that I could feel my face burn as I walked up to the glowing, white hot coals.

Even with my trust in the instructors, I was nervous. I stood there next to Lori as we waited our turn. Then, hand in hand, she and I quickly walked across the bed of fire with bare feet. I didn't need to be reminded not to slow down. If anything, I walked so quickly that my feet barely touched the ground. Maybe that was the secret! As I stepped onto the grass on the other side, my feet did feel somewhat tender. I picked them up, one at a time, to look at the soles. Wondering all the time if I was going to see blisters, or raw flesh. There was hardly any evidence of what I had just done. A couple of spots were just the slightest bit tender. No blisters, no broken skin, and no other evidence of having just walked across those coals. The same for Lori. We looked at each other and started laughing. Probably more from relief than anything else.

I don't think I told anyone, ahead of time, that we were going to do that. I knew most anyone would have thought I was totally nuts. Especially anyone who knew about the balance problems I was having. Just think if I had fallen, halfway across. The results would not have been pretty. But I did it and, in the process, jumpstarted my MS recovery process. It was a good lesson about what goes on in the mind. Every action you take is preceded by a thought, consciously or not. Being afraid of seriously burning my feet would pretty much have insured that I did or stopped me from doing it at all. Believing that I could do it without burning my feet allowed me to do just that.

We often hear "I'll believe it when I see it." That experience was my introduction to the reverse. "I'll see it when I believe it." It was much later when I actually heard that phrase voiced, but the concept was firmly planted way back then. When we were being given instructions to do the "fire walking," we were told, "When you get up there, if you don't believe you can do this without burning your feet, don't do it." The instructor who had once burned her feet confessed that she had not followed that instruction.

As the line waiting to walk across the coals grew shorter, they said anyone who wanted to do it again was welcome. Periodically, they would freshen the coals with a rake and they would glow brightly. Lori and I glanced at each other and got in line. Before we stopped, we had walked across those coals four or five times. We held hands each time, probably for moral support and, also, to make sure that I kept my balance. Words cannot really describe the exhilaration that I felt or the power that seemed to flow through me.

"Believing is seeing" was real for me. Through my long journey with multiple sclerosis, that concept became an integral part of who I am.

Without taking any medication for multiple sclerosis, I did more than slow the progression of the disease. I did, in fact, reverse it. My symptoms slowly disappeared. My body responded to a long, steady regimen of conditioning. Today, no one who didn't know me before would guess that I ever had MS.

Unity church was a blessing to me in many ways. Working with those young people was, itself, a life altering experience. I made many new friends and met many new teachers. They really do "appear when the student is ready." I was exposed to a relatively new concept for me. Not new, I guess, just buried.

I am in charge of my life and everything in it. I don't always understand why I make certain decisions, or I may not understand the "why" of everything that happens with me. What I do know, however, is that whatever I create in my life always starts with a thought in my mind. This was particularly true with my healing process. We forget that our bodies are God's creations and often times capable of healing themselves.

Knowing this allows me to accept responsibility for my life and everything in it. This was a novel concept for me. It is so easy to blame or to hold someone else responsible. But, acknowledging that I am in charge is really a freeing experience.

If I am really responsible for what goes on in my life, then I can do something about what goes on in my life. No more of "there is nothing I can do about it." If *I* did this to me, then *I* can undo it. And while I don't think instantaneous healing is out of the question, I didn't labor under any such illusions about my situation. I spent over forty years getting here. I did not expect to reverse it overnight.

I was continuously exposed to new books. Many of them dealt with these issues. My newly found church was constantly having authors speak. Some would do workshops, as well. Many of them are quite well known today. Some have made appearances for varying lengths of time on the *New York Times Bestseller's List* and on National television talk shows. They have affected millions.

These books with concepts that were, in large part, new to me had a profound effect on my thinking and on my life. If I am stuck in believing that someone did this to me, or that it just happened, then how can I heal myself? How can I undo what someone else did to me? The more I studied the life and words of Jesus, the more clear it was. "Whatever I can do, you can do." These were not idle statements. They were the words of perhaps the greatest teacher ever to walk the face of the earth. It all began to make sense to me.

During the first year after diagnosis, I stayed busy learning as much as I could about multiple sclerosis. A great deal more has been written on the subject today. With all the research that has gone on, the message today is still much the same as it was eighteen years ago. "Finding a cure is just around the corner." I don't think we are any closer to a cure now than we were then.

Early in this process, when I heard about someone with the disease, I often would call and talk about their experiences. I strongly encourage you to do this. The internet and the great strides in communication made by the "social media" make this much easier today.

I came across an article in a magazine about the vice-president of a large mid-western university who resigned from her job a year after beginning to experience symptoms. Her multiple sclerosis had progressed rapidly. At the end of the article was a phone number to call in Cleveland where she was living. I called, thinking someone else would answer. Much to my surprise, she answered the phone. Another "angel" who had a significant impact on my life. Another "teacher who appeared."

She had a gift shop that she opened after having to give up her job at the university. She told me about the terrible deterioration of her body. Then she said if I could see her today, I would have no idea that she ever had MS. She told me about the snowstorm that had hit Cleveland the day before. She had spent all morning shoveling snow for her next door neighbors who were too elderly to do it for themselves.

After listening to her story, I asked, "To what do you attribute your recovery?" She hesitated before she asked, "Do you believe in God?" I said, "Yes, but why do you ask that?" She, quite candidly, told me that some people are offended, or unimpressed with what she has to say and she saw no point in discussing the truth if a person is not ready to hear it.

She told me about her very simple prayer, "Whenever You are ready, would You please take this away from me?" I adopted that prayer as my own and added to it, "In the meantime, would You please assist me in knowing what I need to do." Shortly after that, Dr. Van Sickle told me to start walking. God has many messengers. I firmly believe that wishes come with the power to make them come true. Effort may be required but those wishes don't just happen. We need to pay attention so that we don't miss the message.

From the beginning, I was constantly reading, and searching the web, looking for any information on the disease. One of the books that I read in the first year I attended my new church was, "Myrtle Fillmore, Mother of Unity." She suffered from tuberculosis and by 1886, in her forties, she had been told she had a very short time to live.

Medical treatment at the time offered no hope for a cure. Rather than continuing to place her hopes on existing medicine, she took charge of her own health. She set aside one room in her house where she would sit for hours every day. In the room, she placed a chair for her and a chair for God. She would talk to the different parts of her body, asking them to respond. Two years later, she was disease free. Her faith had been unwavering throughout this process.

Eventually, she went back to her doctors, who had given her such a dismal prognosis. Myrtle was probably less surprised than anyone.

There were no signs of tuberculosis, which at the time was not treatable. She died about fifty years later, in her nineties.

Myrtle's husband Charles, whose faith was not as strong as hers, watched her very intently throughout her healing process. He then had his own healing experience. He had a severe physical handicap since he was ten years old. He had suffered a severe fall and had badly broken one leg. That leg ended up much shorter than the other. He had worn a shoe lift ever since. The difference in the length of his legs was about four inches, because his leg withered as he grew older.

He knew what he had witnessed with Myrtle, and this prompted him into action. He spent hours in that same room, talking to his body and specifically to his damaged leg. After a time, he watched as the leg filled out with muscle, growing stronger every day. Why does this seem so strange? Every movement of the body is preceded by a thought. We need to pay attention.

Myrtle and Charles studied a great deal during this process and started the Unity movement in the years that followed. Today, there are approximately a thousand Unity churches in the United States. Many people over the years have known it as "the healing church," acknowledging the early days. It has been that for me as I learned to apply the principles that have been passed down for so long. We have a great deal of power over what happens to our bodies … are we willing to do the necessary work?

Faith moves mountains, but you have to keep pushing while you are praying.
-- Mason Cooley

The last of the human freedoms is to choose one's attitudes. *– Victor Frankl*

A diamond is just a piece of charcoal that handled stress exceptionally well.
– Anonymous

Chapter 8

Trip to the Top
(Exercise and Walking)

You are never given a wish without also being given the power to make it become true. You may have to work for it however.   *-- Richard Bach*

Once diagnosed with MS, it is never too early to start rehabilitation. Your condition a year from now depends greatly on what you spend the next year doing. To have been diagnosed with multiple sclerosis means that you have already been suffering symptoms of the disease.

These symptoms range from slight irritants to very debilitating effects of the disease. The time to start steady, continuous rehabilitation efforts is at the time you and your doctors have determined the diagnosis, or before.

One of the defining moments in my recovery came soon after my diagnosis by Dr. Maitland. This came after various tests and the elimination of other possible causes of the symptoms. I had a visit with my primary care doctor, Chris Van Sickle, M.D., after that diagnosis.

A recommendation he made to me still rings in my ears almost two decades later. I never had more important advice given to me about the treatment of my MS. He said, "I want you to listen carefully to what I am about to tell you. I want you to walk three or four times a week and I want you to walk at least thirty minutes each time. If you don't do that, you will wake up one morning and not be able to get out of bed. When that happens, you will not walk again."

The advice was not exaggerated. I have experienced what can happen and know that it can be a very crippling disease. I took that advice to heart and started walking. Don't ever forget that it is the failure to start that stops most people.

I couldn't walk more than a hundred and fifty feet at the time, without stopping to rest. I couldn't walk down one side of the mall, a half mile, for many months. I would be exhausted but I would walk anyway. Years later I walked over seventeen miles without stopping once to rest.

Faith and action together are powerful. Think of what happens when you pour water into concrete mix. The combination is far stronger than either of the ingredients. What "happens" to us is not nearly as important as our reaction to it.

For me, physical rehabilitation was largely walking. It was eventually accompanied by many hours in a fitness center doing light exercises over a period of several years. I also did exercises, including light weights, at home. I highly recommend a regular workout routine of walking and light weights as a part of the recovery process. Make it the most important part of your day, along with a regular routine of prayer and meditation.

You do not have to spend all day in the gym. What you do have to do is to set up a regular routine that works for you, at home or in the gym. No matter how good the routine is that you develop, it only works if you do it. You have to take time to take care of yourself now! The alternative is to have the time taken from you later.

My daily routine, for several years now, is a three mile walk and a 30-45 minute workout in the gym with light weights. That takes two hours of my day. That seems like a lot to many people. It doesn't have to be that long. Remember, I was recovering from a very long, debilitating disease. It can be an hour a day or it can be lots of fifteen minute breaks throughout your sixteen waking hours. Rest is important. Exercise is essential. Prayer makes it all come together.

I won't even attempt to list all the benefits of exercising. I will only say that you can spend the two hours each day maintaining your health or, spend it later recovering from health problems. You can choose but, one or the other is likely to happen for most people.

Keep in mind that fatigue is a major symptom of this disease. It stops many people from engaging in the very process, exercise, that offers real hope. Picture this. A good high school athlete goes to school all day; works several hours after school; is too tired to practice and condition his body but, shows up on Friday evening to suit up for his high school football game. Not very realistic if he really wants to play football, is it?

It is about as realistic as letting the fatigue of multiple sclerosis stop you from rehabilitating your body, and expecting to get better anyway.

Your body will either get stronger, or it will get weaker. It will not stay the same. The more you engage in active physical conditioning, the stronger you will get. The less time you spend doing this, the weaker you will get. And yet, I still hear intelligent people saying, "I'm just too exhausted." The result is obvious. The body grows weaker and the fatigue is more pronounced. I even read in material from the National Multiple Sclerosis Society that if you start to feel fatigued that you should rest.

Any athlete, while preparing for competition, becomes exhausted and suffers great fatigue. What happens if they let this exhaustion stop them? The same thing happens to a person with MS who elects not to suffer through this exhaustion. They don't just not get stronger, they get weaker. This is basic; fundamental; elementary; grade school stuff!

The amount of fatigue differs from person to person. I never had "pain," as such, with my MS, as some people do. My body just hurt, and ached. Enough to make me wonder how long I could function. The fatigue is what threatened to stop me. But I would always hear Dr. Van Sickle saying to me, "Walk! Or one day you will wake up and not be able to walk!"

I walked, not three or four times a week as Dr. Van Sickle had recommended, but every day. I knew how addictive behavior could become. And I knew what would happen if I started skipping days. If I missed a day, it was too easy to miss another day, and another, and ... Dr. Van Sickle's warning was always there. "If you like being able to walk, you had better keep walking." That advice was hard to misinterpret.

Walking quickly became the centerpiece of my rehabilitation. Initially, I walked out in the country, on a dirt road that went by my house. I was walking there one day when I had the feeling one gets when realizing that someone is staring at them. I looked up and froze in my tracks. I was looking at the biggest Rottweiler I had ever seen. To this day, I have never seen another one that large.

He was sitting there, in the middle of the road, very erect, like a sentry. Instinctively, I knew not to run. On each side of the road was a barbed wire fence. Neither fence would have stopped him. Besides, he could have gotten to me before I reached either one.

Instead, I just dropped to my knees and held out my hand. He stared for a few seconds, seemed like forever, stood up, trotted over and started licking my hand. About that time, I heard a shriek as the dog's owner discovered where her dog was. She came racing, in a panic, as she apologized profusely. She said she didn't know the dog was out. They "always" kept him inside because of his overly protective, nasty temperament.

After that, I soon began walking in the Tallahassee Mall. It was air conditioned. I didn't have to worry about the heat, the cold, the rain, or the dogs barking and nipping at my heels. I would walk early in the day because a few minutes in the outside heat just drained my energy. As soon as I started going to the Mall, I discovered a door that was left open so that shop employees could get into the stores early in the morning. Early morning walkers, like myself, learned which door to use. Where there is a will, there is a way.

When I started walking there, I could barely make it from the front door to a section where the fountains were located at the time. This probably wasn't even one hundred and fifty feet. I would have to sit down there and rest. After a few minutes, I would get up and walk again, about the same distance. Then I would sit and rest again. Periodically, I would increase my distance. About eighteen months later, I realized I had just walked around the entire mall without stopping. Using layouts of the mall, I calculated the distance to be about one mile. What a milestone that was for me. From less than one hundred and fifty feet to one mile. It wasn't immediate but it was really gratifying.

One day, as I neared the completion of my walk around the Mall, a uniformed deputy sheriff stopped me. This was a bit unsettling, to say the least. I'm sure he could see the question on my face as he immediately explained. "A lady stopped me," he said, "and told me that you were drunk. I had to make sure that you were okay." He was very calm and courteous as he explained why he had stopped me. That is, until I explained to him why my walk was so unsteady and erratic. I smiled as I said, "I only wish that I was drunk." "What do you mean?" he asked. I very calmly answered, "The reason that I walk like I am drunk is that I have multiple sclerosis. That is why I am in here walking to begin with."

To say that he was caught totally by surprise would be an understatement. His face turned beet red as he absorbed what I had said. He was visibly embarrassed as he said, "Please accept my apologies. And I will explain to her." I must admit, I felt some degree of satisfaction at seeing how embarrassed he was. I had this thought that maybe she would be just as embarrassed as the policeman had been. And I realized that what they did was quite natural and quite admirable. I appeared to be drunk. They were doing what they needed to do, for me. I remembered the day I lay on the ground in the park for hours with no one bothering to check on me.

Each time, before I finished walking, a battle would ensue within. Fatigue was always the competition. "I am just too exhausted." And right behind that I would hear, "If you like walking, you better keep walking." Eventually I got to the point that I knew. Really knew! I had to keep walking if I wanted to be able to walk. "Use it or, lose it." Use the fatigue as a signal to walk, not as a signal to rest.

Sometime later, my brother Jerry gave me a membership to a local gym. Jerry had been walking for quite a while, having been a jogger for years. He walked often and worked out regularly, a good role model. In retrospect, my initial workout routine was not very ambitious. I would go two or three times a week and would spend most of my time on the treadmill. This helped to establish my walking routine and became an integral part of my conditioning.

My mother was a real inspiration to me. She would routinely walk several miles each day. She did this for many years. There were many weeks when she would walk 60 miles a week. Only in the last couple of years, as her knees have bothered her so much, has she begun to walk less. There are days she can't even walk a quarter of a mile because of pain in her knees. Then, there are days when she will walk several miles. She doesn't do this all at once. She may walk a couple of miles before breakfast, a couple of miles after breakfast, and continue on that pace all day long some days. She would walk 10 or 12 miles a day well into her eighties. My 88 year old mother is still an exceptional athlete, constantly pushing herself.

Eventually, I began walking in grocery stores. There was always a convenient one nearby and I didn't walk in the same one all of the time, or at their busiest times. I preferred walking there because I liked seeing more people. I kept my walking shoes in my car and I would stop at a grocery store, wherever I happened to be, and do my walking. By then, I was walking two miles each day.

When I went back to work, after not having worked for three years because of my MS, I noticed very quickly that working eight hours in a day would tire me out. I simply didn't feel like doing anything by the time I got home.

I would lie down and go to sleep. Of course, it was difficult to get up hours later and walk. Often, I would end up not walking. I knew that I had to correct this and I made a new rule for myself. When I left work, I would walk for two miles before I went home. I quickly realized that after walking for two miles, I didn't feel like going to bed until hours later. I would come home and have lots of extra time to do whatever I felt like doing instead of going to bed and sleeping.

It did not matter that I was tired. If I kept walking, the exhaustion turned into what I call "a good tired." And this would be accompanied by lots of energy. I came to understand the meaning of "a runner's high." No longer did I go home and "crash." Nor did I want to. Instead of "crashing," I would spend the next few hours constructively. It greatly lengthened my days and I slowly felt myself getting stronger in the process.

I noticed over time that walking regularly would give me encouragement. Each time would be slightly easier. Walking two miles became routine. If I failed to walk for even one day, I missed it. I would be conscious of an empty feeling inside, followed by an irritable feeling. I would get tired much more quickly than if I had walked.

I am reminded of a co-worker who decided, in his fifties, to be a sprinter on a competitive basis. He didn't just go out the next day and do it. He started to train. He would work all day, in a stressful job, and then go to the track and run sprints. Hard to imagine?

Just think of all he accomplished by doing that. In addition to improving the general health of his body, he relieved the stress which was ever present in his job. The psychological benefits cannot even be measured.

Eventually, he ran so well in the state competition that he qualified for the nationals in his age group. There he qualified to compete internationally in his age group. This, from a man who began his racing career in his late fifties. At the international event in Spain, he placed eighth. Think of it. In his age group, he was clocked as being the eighth fastest man in the world.

He is one of the many inspirational people to enter my life over the years. He didn't stop there, however. A year later, after having continued training, he went to the state competition and set a state record for his age group in the one hundred meter dash. He missed setting a state record by a fraction of a second in the two hundred meter race

This was an inspiration to me and an important one. Here was a man now sixty who started running competitively in his mid-fifties. Yet, he decided that he wanted to do this. It would have been impressive if he had been a sprinter in his teens and twenties. Retraining the muscles to do what they have done before, at his age, would have been an accomplishment. But, to start training in his fifties to be a sprinter is remarkable. To become the fastest sixty year old man to ever run the 100 meter race in Florida is nothing short of incredible.

Anyone could have looked at his life and marveled at his success. Married to his high school sweetheart, the father of three successful children was nearing retirement age where he had served in a management position over twenty years.

No one would have expected him to put in the hours he did, training to be a competitive sprinter. Can you imagine the hours of training when he was already tired from working? Not that raising three teenagers is an easy task. Can you imagine the pain of forcing a body already in its late-fifties down a track at that speed? He could see it, and he believed it.

What does that have to do with multiple sclerosis?

From barely being able to walk because of my MS, I walked with a cane for years. I walked thousands of miles, eventually walking seventeen miles without so much as stopping once to rest. The "yes but" is still there for some. It is "yes, but MS affects different people differently."

I totally agree that different people are affected differently. I also know that I could have just stayed home and rested all of these days. And there were many days that I was simply too tired to walk. Too fatigued – after all, this symptom is common to people who have MS. When an athlete trains, there may be days or hours following a hard workout when the athlete feels fatigued.

One of the primary symptoms of MS is fatigue. It adversely affected me greatly for years. It was from sheer will that I forced myself to walk those two miles every day. My body would sometimes hurt, literally ache, as I was walking. It really was a test of my willpower and my endurance. The grocery store was a great place to walk, and still is. I would walk up and down those aisles until I had walked my two miles. The stores are clean, well-lighted, pleasant places to shop, or walk. I made a rule that I couldn't shop until I walked. Too easy to get distracted.

For a while, I was frequently asked by store employees if they could help me find something. I was somewhat uneasy that someone would decide they didn't want me in there walking. Every single employee, however, was always friendly and helpful to me. I would explain that I was "just" walking, and it wasn't long before most of the employees knew what I was doing.

I have done that for years and have met and talked to many store employees and customers. It has been a great way to meet people and make walking a more fun way to exercise.

In Tallahassee, there are several 5-K races that are run at the same times each year. One day I was prompted to walk in one of these races, just to see if I could finish. I realized that I had to get in better condition before attempting this. So, instead of walking two miles each day, I began walking three miles each day, just to make sure I would be able to finish. My first race was really an interesting one for me in many respects. I discovered that walking on a treadmill in an air conditioned gym or walking in an air conditioned grocery store was somewhat different from walking three miles cross-country, or on an outside track. That first 5-K race, I finished dead last. That means last, and almost "dead." I forget how many people were in that race but, I do remember that I was the last one to finish.

For the last mile, I wanted so badly to quit; to sit down and rest. But, I was determined to finish. When I was less than a hundred yards from the finish line, I struggled as I came down the stretch. Two ladies on the race staff noticed me approaching and that I was staggering. They quickly came out to make sure that I was OK. I was probably fifty yards away when they met me.

They walked with me, one on each side. I explained to them that I had multiple sclerosis and this was the first time I had ever done a 5-K race. I added that I was feeling very fatigued, but wanted to finish. They walked the rest of the way with me. Before we got to the finish line, one of them pointed out a shortcut that would get us to the finish line much quicker. I simply smiled and said, "I am this close and I really want to finish." We walked the rest of the way. I've always remembered their kindness.

This illustrates something that is so important to remember for anyone involved with a person with a disability. The best thing that can be done to assist that person is to enable them to function. "Taking care of them" may be something you want to do, and not what is necessarily best for them.

Give a man a fish and he eats for a day; teach a man to fish and he eats for a life time. **--Chinese Proverb**

Assisting them in learning to take care of themselves is helpful. Insisting that they are not capable is harmful. Remember to empower, not to disable, them.

That was the first 5-K race that I did. I kept training harder and harder, so when it was time for the next 5-K, I was better prepared. I was not the last person to finish. Between 20 and 30 people finished behind me. That number increased each time that I did a 5-K race after that.

Finally, I realized how time-consuming these races were for me. I would go out early on a Saturday morning to get registered. After we did the race, the awards were presented. I had spent half a day doing a three mile race by the time I got back home.

Time had become very important to me by then … that can happen as we age. I could spend five minutes going to a store near me, walk three miles in an hour, and be back home in a few minutes. It didn't take nearly as much of my time as going to compete in a full-fledged race, and I still got to do my walking.

I did miss all of the excitement involved in being at a race with all of those people. Even people who were not as well conditioned as I, were out there walking and having fun. It was a great atmosphere. I really appreciate all of the people who stay involved in organizing and promoting those races. What a great service they provide. The Gulf Winds Track Club in Tallahassee really helps to crystalize the importance of running and walking in achieving and maintaining overall health. I have continued my walking inside and my standard has become three miles a day. This takes me about an hour.

For a time, I considered walking a marathon. It was another goal for me. As a result, I began to slowly increase the distance I walked each day. I had gotten to where I would often walk 6 or 7 miles when I had time. So, I decided to push it. I walked over seventeen miles in a store one Saturday, without stopping to rest once. That is when I realized I really could train enough to walk a marathon. The urge, however, had passed.

I wanted to continue conditioning. I just didn't need to condition myself to do a marathon. Three miles a day was good for me. I have walked three miles a day, seven days a week, for many years. I have walked well over eight thousand miles during that time. I am in far better condition than I would have been otherwise.

My objective was to keep myself walking. There is no question in my mind that it has greatly improved my general conditioning as well as the effect that MS has had on my life. I can never thank Dr. Van Sickle enough for the advice he gave me, "If you want to keep walking, walk." I see him occasionally in the store as I "keep walking" almost two decades later.

As I continued my walking, my symptoms improved and disappeared. I haven't forgotten those times when my symptoms so greatly interfered with my everyday activities, including my walking and my ability to hold a job.

After not being able to work for three years, I re-joined the work force and worked many more years before ultimately retiring. I have continued my walking and working out. I don't work out less, I do even more. I didn't retire to quit. I retired to go back to school. I chose, instead, to write this book.

You can do what I have done. It takes hard work, faith, and determination. In the next chapter we take a look at how the pharmaceuticals continue to profit from our misery while reporting huge profits selling drugs that are supposed to improve symptoms.

The future depends on what we do in the present. — *Gandhi*

It's the start that stops most people.
—*Don Shula*

Chapter 9

Just Around the Corner
(Doctors and Pharmaceuticals)

One of the first duties of a physician is to educate the masses not to take medicine.
-- William Oster

I first saw a neurologist in December of 1992, having been referred there by my general practitioner. Over the next couple of years, I was diagnosed with multiple sclerosis. I remember reading back then that "a cure is just around the corner." I felt relief, hope, and excitement. Maybe this would not last too long. Eighteen years later, I was reading in a publication put out by the National Multiple Sclerosis Society that "a cure is just around the corner." Having grown accustomed to the pharmaceutical marketing machine, it is hard to visualize what this "corner" may look like. Maybe something like a trip to Mars on a pack mule.

The simple truth? "Treating" symptoms is far more profitable than a cure would be. Their primary objective is to make money. Curing patients is secondary.

Some doctors like to play God. They have little training in this area. In general, they do the best they can with the training they have and with the medicines that are available to them. Many doctors stay too busy to allow time to learn about all of the medicines they are prescribing. They rely heavily on the sales representatives of the pharmaceutical companies to advise them on the available medicines. This is appalling. Those people are not doctors. Much of their knowledge comes from their employers, the pharmaceutical companies. Their success depends on how successful they are in selling their products to the doctors; NOT how successful the doctors are in healing their patients. Does anyone see anything remotely wrong with this system?

Over the years, I have been blessed to have some really good doctors. However, not all doctors fall into that category. Not everyone, of any profession, is among the best. A common perception among many, if not most, Americans is that we get the best medical care available in the world. This also assumes that the medical training our doctors receive here, is the best available. Neither is necessarily true.

All medical schools within this country are certainly not of the same quality. It is safe to assume the same is true worldwide. This notion of superior medical treatment in this country is pure arrogance on our part. We consider ourselves to be so advanced that we fail to see reality. We don't notice the serious decline in our educational system nor the control exerted by the pharmaceutical companies over the entire health care system.

Sometimes the best a doctor can do is to not harm the patient. They need to forget about being a scientist and just help nature as best they can.

People from around the world come to this country for medical treatment. People leave this country for the same reason. The number of patients who die in hospitals in this country, as a result of treatment received while there, is simply staggering. The workload of doctors in residency is glorified in television and movies. Naturally, much of this fiction is based on fact. Is it any wonder that mistakes are made and people die unnecessarily?

ABC World News reported in July of 2011 about a study from the Journal of General Internal Medicine. This study showed that counties with teaching hospitals reported a ten percent increase in deaths from medication errors in July. That correlates with an influx of inexperienced residents trying to learn a new system while working 36 hour shifts. And this is the world's greatest health care system. Sounds more like fraternity hazing. The interns are forced to play Russian roulette with the lives of patients. Whatever happened to the Hippocratic tradition of "First, do no harm?" The system makes this a joke. We have eight hour workdays. Why do we routinely require more from people who literally hold lives in their hands? Now, we have too many doctors and administrators in the system who don't seem to remember, understand or respect this code.

The treatment of multiple sclerosis is typical of today's medicine. The disease has been named for over a century. There is no cure, and none in sight. But "just around the corner," there may be hope. Treatment, after over 100 years, still consists of several questionable attempts to fight the symptoms. With some patients, these symptoms are mild. With others, they are severe. They are present in different combinations and are debilitating, in varying degrees.

Corticosteroids may be the most common of treatments given to MS patients. It reduces inflammation that spikes during a relapse. It may be taken orally or intra-venously. As a word of caution to diabetics, it sometimes causes a spike in blood sugar levels and, sometimes, to very dangerous levels. I had one such treatment and ended up with blood sugar exceeding 600, when it should be around 100. I didn't do that anymore.

Interferons, such as Betaseron, Avonex and Rebif are thought by some to slow the rate at which multiple sclerosis symptoms worsen. How anyone can even begin to make this assertion has always puzzled me. Start from the place of general agreement about MS.

There are a large number of symptoms, and people have them in different combinations. Relapse rates vary greatly. Given this myriad of possibilities, how does anyone possibly know that after taking the medication, my relapse rate will be less than it would have been without the medication? I know of no way to determine that or to accurately predict the course of the disease in anyone. From my extensive reading over two decades, I am not aware that anyone else knows either. Along with this lack of knowledge, HOWEVER, we do know interferons can cause serious liver damage.

Glatiramer, or copaxone, is "believed" by doctors to work by blocking the immune system's attack on myelin. It is taken subcutaneously (under the skin) once daily. Flushing and shortness of breath are often experienced after injection. If you knew of nothing wrong and began flushing and had difficulty breathing, would it occur to you that something was wrong? And you take this medicine why? Because the drug companies profit from your taking it and told the doctors it "may" have some positive effect on your MS. Does "herd of sheep" ring a bell?

Natalizumab, or Tysabri, is designed to work by interfering with the movement of potentially damaging immune cells from the bloodstream to the brain and spinal cord. It is, generally, reserved for people who see no results from, or can't tolerate, other kinds of treatment. This is BECAUSE Tysabri increases the risk of progressive multifocal leuko-encephalopathy, a brain infection that is usually fatal. Do you hear me? It increases the risk of death. A friend of mine, when starting a new medicine said to me, "What do I have to lose?"

Mitoxantrone, known as Novantrone, is an immunosuppressant drug. Mostly, it is used in people who have advanced multiple sclerosis. It can be harmful to the heart. Why risk killing someone? Assisted suicides generally are not legal. Giving medicine to MS patients that may hasten their death is somehow okay.

Some medicines have been abandoned along the way ... some because they were not effective and some because the side effects were simply too heavy a price to pay. Given that, let us look at the side effects of the remaining medicines discussed above. Give some thought to when treatments are worse than the disease. When are the risks greater than the reward?

One of the five medicines is extremely dangerous for diabetics. One can cause serious liver damage. One may cause blushing and shortness of breath after injection. One increases the risk of a brain infection that is usually fatal. One can be so harmful to the heart that it is only used in very advanced cases of MS. So let me ask, "Why do we make assisted suicide a crime while we allow the pharmaceutical company to provide, and a doctor to administer, a medicine that may have the same result?" Some make the argument that the motive is different even though the result may be the same. Does this motive change the result?

A man is rushing his pregnant wife to the hospital. He runs a red light causing an accident that kills the other driver. Does it really matter that his motive was just to get his wife to the hospital? The obvious primary motive for the pharmaceutical company is not saving lives. It is profitability.

Most people would be amazed to learn that the profitability of our big pharmaceutical companies compares very favorably to that of the big oil companies.

I was fortunate to never start taking any medication for multiple sclerosis. It wasn't that I was in any way opposed to medicines in general. At one time, I was taking fifteen prescription medications. I now take four. With the many different side effects associated with so many drugs, I was simply not inclined to be a guinea pig for our drug industry. If you think that the Food and Drug Administration (FDA) is only motivated by its purpose to protect the public as it was intended to do, you are somewhat misinformed. The drug companies historically have provided a huge portion of the FDA's budget. They pay huge fees to get their medicines approved. But surely you don't believe that money would influence actions of the FDA?

Do the math. The pharmaceuticals have an unending, growing stream of income from selling drugs that do not even purport to cure multiple sclerosis. The cost to the patients for some of this medicine is exorbitant. In some cases, patients pay thousands of dollars per year for one medicine. They don't expect to be cured, just "helped." There is no medication that is known to cure MS. So, what we have is a pharmaceutical industry that provides "helping" medicines to a half million people with a terrible debilitating disease. These medicines "may" help patients. "Why" is unknown. Pharmaceutical companies take our money from us because they can. As a society, we condone this. Our government enables it. We pretend that our government protects us. One of the first responsibilities of a doctor should be to warn patients about the possible side effects of a medication. As Benjamin Franklin noted, "God heals and the doctor takes the fees."

The problem is not limited to patients with MS, of course. A study released by the Kaiser Family Foundation in 2006, showed that the number of prescriptions written in this country every year is sufficient to supply every man, woman and child with almost 13 prescription drugs. This doesn't even consider all of the over-the-counter drugs that patients take on their own.

This study showed that the number of prescriptions for drugs per person in this country had increased by 62% in twelve years. In many cases we do not even know how these drugs react when used together.

In the field of psychiatry alone, we have seen a huge shift away from face to face therapy. The shift to treatment with pharmaceuticals has become more prevalent. This is a classic case of treating the symptoms, rather than the "disease." What it does accomplish is to greatly increase the number of patients that a doctor can treat simultaneously.

We keep them medicated. A great doctor suggested that the greatest difference between man and animals is man's great propensity to take medicine.

In 2008, a nationwide survey done by Qato, et al, and published in the *Journal of the American Medical Association*, showed that 29 percent of people in this country used at least five prescription medications at the same time. Only three years before, an article in *Medscape* said seventeen percent took three or more simultaneously. Studies have shown an increase, by sixty-five percent, in hospitalizations or death caused by overdoses of prescription medications in the past seven years.

Parents of most children would probably be amazed to find out that few drugs are ever tested on infants. Close to eighty percent of children in hospitals are given medications that have never been approved to be given to children. A survey done in 1999 in England showed that ninety percent of infants were prescribed medicines that were never approved for safety or effectiveness in children. As one might expect, drug reactions in children given unapproved medicine is several times higher than that of medicine which has been approved.

Why is such callous disregard for the health and lives of infants permitted in modern hospitals? Who is to blame? Is it the parents? Is it the doctors? Hospitals? Or pharmaceutical companies? Or, is it all four? When is it appropriate for law enforcement agencies to become involved? I hear of doctors getting into trouble for misusing prescriptions for adults. Quite frankly, I don't recall ever hearing of a doctor being in trouble for prescribing, for infants and children, medicine that has not been approved for their use.

Why does the government, with its rules and laws, force the inoculation of children when there are strong indications that many children are harmed by the vaccines? Just how many inoculations are required for a child to be admitted to school?

The problem is especially serious with our elderly patients, many of whom are on so many medicines that it can't help but affect them, both physically and mentally. Pharmaceutical companies continue to make huge profits and the insurance companies just raise their rates. How often do you hear of either losing money?

People supporting this system seem to ignore statistics which should be alarming to anyone. It is no wonder that the best drugs available to treat MS help so little and have so many side effects. The youngest people, the oldest people, people with multiple sclerosis and the general public, are all treated with the same disregard by pharmaceutical companies. All of these people are, to them, giant streams of income.

Proponents of our current system go out of their way to discredit other methods of treatment. A common criticism is, "Those are not really scientifically proven." As if the usefulness and safety of all medicine is. Medical people work with insurance companies to decide who gets reimbursed and, as you can imagine, the "competition" gets very little. Doctors questioning conventional treatments in favor of alternative ones, will often be subjected to severe criticism and even ridicule from contemporaries for directing patients to unconventional treatments. All of this in spite of the fact that whatever is totally accepted as normal treatment today, may be considered as ineffective, or even dangerous, ten years from now.

The reality is that Eastern medicine, like acupuncture, has been practiced for centuries in other parts of the world. It produces some amazing results. Western medicine did not cure, or even significantly improve, my very painful carpal tunnel syndrome. More than once, the pain was so bad that I wore leather braces on both wrists to keep them straight and alleviate the pain. This was fairly standard procedure, I was told, before considering any surgery.

Keeping my wrists straight helped reduce the pain, but it did nothing to cure the problem. This is typical much of the time with Western medicine. I had a couple of acupuncture treatments and my pain disappeared. Years later, it has not returned again. I wouldn't even have known to try that except a co-worker told me that acupuncture had solved that problem for her. A friend of mine had surgery for the same thing, on one wrist, at a cost of ten thousand dollars. Common practice!

How many doctors allow patients to suffer incredible pain, or simply prescribe pain medication when acupuncture has been so successful at alleviating pain? How many doctors simply prescribe medication for pain rather than looking for the cause of the pain and treating that?

Think about it. If you have pain, do you simply want medication to mask the pain, or do you want the doctor to determine the cause of the pain and stop it? If you have kidney stones, do you want the stones dissolved or removed? Or, do you simply want medication to mask the pain caused by the stone tearing through your body? If you have appendicitis, do you want your appendix removed, or do you want some medicine to mask the fact that your appendix is about to burst?

In the late 1800's and early 1900's, the *American Medical Association* had a clause in its code of ethics that members were not allowed to consult with any medical doctor who also practiced homeopathy. Nor were doctors allowed to treat such a doctor's patients. It was okay for doctors to "bleed" their patients to death during this same period, or to prescribe mercury and other such agents to patients. Yet, consulting with a homeopath was "criminal."

In addition to being very territorial, doctors simply do not have the time, or take the time, to research medicines as the pharmaceutical companies are supposed to be doing. They have the right to rely on an FDA approval for a drug; that it is safe and does what it is advertised to do. Except, this reliance has been proven over and over again not to be warranted. What does that knowledge do to a doctor's responsibility?

Doctors rely on the pharmaceutical salesmen to tell them about new drugs and what these drugs are designed to do. This is an over simplification, of course, because many doctors are diligent and take their oath seriously. If a governmental agency approves a medicine, shouldn't we be able to rely on that approval? The truth is that the public should be very skeptical ... of the FDA, of any drug going into their bodies, and of any politician accepting money from drug companies.

To get a realistic view of our pharmaceutical industry, one need only look to see the small number of drugs that survive thirty years or more. They know what they are doing and that would not be profitable. Patents on drugs only last so long and the pharmaceutical industry has a decided financial interest in having "new" ones as the patents expire.

They have a huge market supplying drugs to treat different symptoms of the disease. They make billions.

Nine years ago, the combined profits of the ten largest pharmaceutical companies was greater than the combined profits of the remaining 490 companies in the Fortune 500. This startling revelation was made in a book, *The Truth about Drug Companies*, by Marcia Angell, M.D., and published by Random House. The only reason this has not remained true is because of the outrageous profits made by the oil companies and arms manufacturers during our Middle Eastern wars. You think foreign policy decisions are not affected by money from those companies and their lobbyists?

In an article in *Skeptical Inquirer* in the summer of 2006, this same Marcia Angell, M.D., wrote the following: "Over the past two decades the pharmaceutical industry has moved very far from its original high purpose of discovering and producing useful new drugs. Now primarily a marketing machine to sell drugs of dubious benefit, this industry uses its wealth and power to co-opt every institution that might stand in its way, including the U.S. Congress, the FDA, academic medical centers, and the medical profession itself." This doctor has earned our attention and our respect. At the time of this statement, she was a Harvard professor and former editor of *The New England Journal of Medicine*. Don't ignore her warnings.

I would take issue with only one statement that Dr. Angell made. It has been going on much longer than two decades. One need only look at the massive inoculation program for Polio in the mid-twentieth century.

Dr. Herbert Ratner, M.D., contributed greatly to the formation of La Leche League when he was Health Commissioner for Oak Park, Illinois. He was even more famous for his part in exposing the polio vaccine scandal which was perpetrated by the drug companies with the cooperation of the FDA. He firmly believed that thousands of children were harmed by the incomplete research and premature distribution of the Salk vaccine.

Polio appeared to go down after the vaccine was introduced. This was because the U.S. Health Service adopted tougher polio reporting requirements. Meningitis was then reported for many cases that would have been reported as polio before, according to an article in *Oak Leaves*, July 6, 2005. He was editor of the *Bulletin of the American Association of Public Health Physicians* when he took on the corrupt polio vaccine establishment. In an editorial in the *Bulletin*, he "questioned the propriety of imposing upon the medical profession at large, and local health officials in particular, an enforced inoculation program without providing the written report on which the program was based. Reports included fraudulent information. The number of patients inoculated with the vaccine who subsequently contracted polio was large. Huge!

"The vaccine was fast tracked through government approval processes with devastating results. The more people that were vaccinated, the more cases of polio surfaced. By 1959, over 300,000,000 doses of vaccine had been administered in the nation. By some estimates, between fifteen and twenty percent of patients with polio were likely to have had three shots." *Journal of American Medical Association*, April 9, 1960.

In May of 1960, Dr. Ratner chaired a panel reviewing the vaccine and the conclusions were reprinted in the *Illinois Medical Journal* in August of 1960. The vaccine was exposed as a "frank and ineptly disguised fraud." Dr. Bernard Greenburg, from that panel, testified at Congressional hearings. He revealed how data had been manipulated to hide the dangers and ineffectiveness of the vaccine. He explained how methodology of reporting was changed to give the perception of an overall reduction in polio cases.

Dr. Ratner stated publicly that in "1957 the largest producers of Salk vaccine had several million dollars' worth of vaccine which did not pass minimum requirements for the U.S. Public Health Service. These were values of fifty years ago!

The Division of Biological Standards reinterpreted its minimum requirements to make possible the utilization of the vaccine. In the February 16, 1961 issue of the *Journal of American Medical Association*, Dr. Ratner denounced the Salk vaccine and said that the 335 million polio shots given by then were a waste because they were too weak to be effective. He went on to say that the shots were no more dependable than if NO vaccination had taken place. Crimes against hundreds of millions of people were committed by the pharmaceutical companies in marketing the Salk vaccine. This fraud was made possible by the government.

Now we annually take flu vaccines provided by these same companies with the same motives. Doctors are willing participants. How do they know the flu vaccines are effective? Yet, they recommend to patients that they get the "flu" shot. Decades ago they recommended to a populace of a quarter of a billion people that they take the polio vaccine which was worthless. A few decades ago, I remember long lines "at the pumps" and gas rationing. We hear those same fears today. What happened in between? People truly are "like cattle." But more intelligent? I wonder

Did anyone go to prison for the massive fraud against a fearful public by the government and the drug companies for the Salk vaccine scandal? The government used our money to support the cover up of the massive fraud committed by the pharmaceutical companies.

In the same way they "bailed out" and covered up the fraud perpetrated on the American people by Wall Street brokers and our bankers. How many hundreds of millions of our tax money went to the "criminals" while most of the economy remains mired in the worst economy since the great depression? Wall Street was well represented among the President's advisors. Starting with the Treasury Secretary, his economic advisors had great connections to "business as usual." The taxpayers will have to repay the hundreds of millions in stimulus money used to save Wall Street. While the country remains mired in a period of high unemployment, Wall Street routinely hands out million dollar bonuses to its own. Who represented the general populace? Only the hapless American voter.

Our entire system is flawed, seriously flawed. We have an FDA set up to protect us. It takes millions upon millions of dollars to get a medicine through our system before it goes to market. It may take years to get final approval. And then we cannot trust their decisions. The same, or similar, medicine may have been on the market in Europe for years. The argument for our system is that it is better to be safe. A pathetic argument at best.

To a cancer patient given a short time to live, it can't make much sense. He/she is told that the treatment which might save his/her life won't be approved for use in this country for a number of years. And all too often, the FDA approves a medication that does untold damage before it is taken off the market.

I started taking a closer look at the medicine I was taking after I read an article in a newsletter years ago. I still remember the name of the article, "*Six drugs that can kill...*" That immediately grabbed my attention. I didn't have to read too far before I discovered that a medication that I had been taking for years, increased the risk of heart attacks by four times. I wasn't told this when I started taking the medicine or at any time during the years I took it. At the time that article was written, research had shown that it was true. I called my doctor's office and said that I wasn't taking the medicine anymore. The story doesn't end there, however.

What followed will give you a better idea of the seriousness of this problem. TWO YEARS after I had stopped the medication, I was watching the CBS evening news one evening. One of the lead stories was an announcement of a new medical discovery. The same drug was discovered to increase the risk of heart attacks by four times. Think about it! Two more years had passed. The news report, of course, did not mention how long this had been known by the drug companies and the regulators. It should be noted the drug companies spend many millions on media advertising.

The drug was taken off the market two years after I stopped taking it, for the very reason that I stopped taking it. When I read about the problem, lots of people knew about it. This included the pharmaceutical company's employees who obviously knew the risk. The FDA knew the risk. For two years after I stopped taking it, the drug company was still marketing an FDA approved drug that increased the likelihood of a heart attack by four times. It was subsequently taken off the market, then allowed back on the market again, at least a couple of times. Three years later they were still fighting to keep it on the market. Today, attorneys are preparing for extensive litigation against the company involved and running ads on TV to alert people who were harmed while taking that drug. The system is broken. It is sick! It is owned and financed by the industry it purports to regulate.

The conspiracy is not simply against MS patients. That is really such a small part of a much larger scandalous situation. It is a scandal that continues unabated in spite of the efforts of people like Dr. Angell. In her writings about the drug companies, she points to the wealth and power of this industry. They control Congress on any issue important to them. They control the FDA, the medical centers, and the medical profession itself. We need to look at the failure of the industry to develop medicines that will cure multiple sclerosis. The failure is attributable to the greed of the pharmaceutical industry as a whole. Multiple sclerosis is such a small part of that never ending, ever growing disaster. Their objective is to maximize their profits. We are simply dollar signs to them.

Great physicians practice and collect their fees for not healing. Decades pass with no cure in sight. The number of patients suffering continues to rise. The pharmaceuticals smile as they make their deposits, growing richer and more powerful by the day.

Their executives are among the highest paid in business. Their sales forces are paid well, as are any politicians who can help them along the way. The media giants get paid well by the huge advertising budgets and are always available for positive news coverage for the companies and for the politicians. As a rule, stockholders get paid well. While profits are incredibly excessive, the consequences of the common use of more than one drug at a time are rarely known.

Many doctors are exceptional. Some medical discoveries are great. However, there are too many exceptions to both of these statements. Who is willing to accept the responsibility?

The *New York Times* uncovered a story that Pfizer admitted to paying twenty million dollars in the last six months of 2009 alone, to 4500 doctors for "consultation" and for speaking on their behalf. This did not even include doctors outside of the U.S. This is 2011. I recently attended a dinner at a nice Tallahassee restaurant, all of which was paid for by a drug company. The attendees were all MS patients.

The speaker was a local neurologist who at least disclosed that he was being paid by the drug company to speak on their behalf. His stated objective was to convince patients that they should be taking one of the available drugs.

Earlier in this chapter, I discussed the drugs available for multiple sclerosis, their efficacy and the known side effects. Can you imagine a more obvious conflict of interest than to have a doctor, paid by the drug company, explain to you why you should be taking one of the drugs they put on the market? Would you be comfortable with your attorney who was "honest" enough to tell you that he was on the payroll of your legal adversary? Of course not. Yet a doctor does the same and that is ethical?

I detected no embarrassment about this blatant conflict. This is worse than pathetic. He obviously failed to see anything unethical about his behavior. Do you understand the scope of your responsibility where your health is involved? Take charge of your health; your body; your life. You cannot change the past. You may not be here tomorrow. Today you can make a difference.

The doctor, if he forgets he is only the assistant to nature and zealously takes over the stage, may so add to what nature is already doing well that he actually throws the patient into shock by the vigour he adds to nature's forces.
-- Herbert Ratner, M.D.

"If you aren't sure about the contents of this chapter, you may want to read it again."

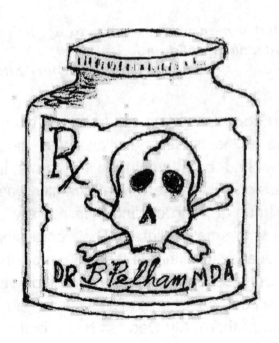

Chapter 10

What a Trip!
(Reflections)

What a man really wishes to do, he will find a means of doing.
>   *-- George Bernard Shaw*

Growing up on a farm in Northwest Florida in the fifties and sixties was hard. My parents had both grown up on farms in the depression. They knew what scarcity was like, as children growing up and then as very young adults with small children. The depression era was not easy for either of them. My mom lived in town on weekends during her senior year in high school so she could have a job at a restaurant there. My Dad left home in the tenth grade and worked in the mills in Western Central Georgia, sending money home to his Mom to help feed the other kids., Like so many in this country in that era, they had a hard life.

Although the world is full of suffering, it is full also of the overcoming of it.
-- Helen Keller

It was hard for my siblings and me growing up. I didn't know how hard at the time. I didn't have anything with which to compare it. Like most people, I was shaped by the early years of my life.

I worked hard on the farm and worked hard to do well in school. I was a workaholic at a very early age. I went to school, came home, worked in the fields and did homework until late at night. The summers were for working longer and harder. It was a stressful life for us all. My father was always pushing us to work harder and do more. He was always worn out himself because all he seemed to be able to do was work hard, and make sure we were doing the same.

My mom worked harder than any of us. She worked in the garden, canned vegetables, worked in the fields, cooked meals, did laundry, had five babies, made clothes for me and my siblings, helped with homework, and took care of all the cuts, scrapes and bruises that we had. She had an alcoholic, workaholic husband, five kids to raise, endless work to get done, and I really don't know how she survived it all.

Along with all of the farm work that had to be done, I was as driven with my work at school as my Dad was with his work on the farm. After school, I worked in the fields until dark; did homework until it was finished, which often was very late; and started the whole thing over with chores before school early the next morning so that I could catch the bus by 7:00 am.

I loved school. There was no physical labor involved. I got positive feedback from my teachers and I loved being around all of my friends. Even then, I was a workaholic. Not only did I demand of myself that I make the best grades, I spent untold hours at recess, lunchtime, and study halls, helping classmates with their homework. I also spent lots of time on extracurricular activities that I could do while at school. There was Student Council, Honor Society and other clubs, along with trying to be a friend to everybody. Staying so busy all of the time at home and at school was stressful.

After graduating from high school, I worked the summer on the farm and started college in September, with barely a break to "catch my breath." At college, I had lots of part-time jobs, needing the money to stay in school. I worked so hard that I missed a lot that was going on. It was an exciting time to be a student and a bit unnerving at the same time. The civil rights movement was in full force. The Viet Nam War was getting bigger with each passing month and fear of getting drafted kept many in school. I was worn out with work and school but really did not want to go to Viet Nam. Some people never returned. Of those who did, many came home badly injured, mentally and physically. Relatively speaking, a few suffered greatly while life went on for most.

I was in the reserves and did not go. That war was hard on the country as a whole and harder on the people who served. Wars are like that and we seem to keep one or more going all of the time. Politicians and the "military/industrial complex" that President Eisenhower warned us about see to that. We kill each other for various reasons. The reason always makes sense to a lot of people; enough to keep the war going. Sometimes it is out of fear. Sometimes it is because of religious differences. Sometimes it is for economic reasons. Sometimes it is just because "someone" needs a war going…

I was married at twenty. I didn't know enough to know that I was too young. We graduated from college and I took a job in Miami. I was back in Tallahassee, in law school, less than a year later. I spent too much time working when I should have been studying or attending classes. After graduating, I kept working in real estate rather than practicing law. I was as much of a workaholic as my Dad had ever been. In the process, I ruined two marriages, relationships with my two daughters, and my health. While my journey with multiple sclerosis is the subject of this book, it was the first of several diseases that I encountered on my journey. My battle with multiple sclerosis was the beginning of a journey that included diabetes, myasthenia gravis, trigeminal neuralgia, arthritis and MRSA staph infection. They all played a part in my battle for health. I will save that discussion for a later time. The lessons on my journey with multiple sclerosis served me quite well in the other battles, all of which I obviously survived.

This book has been written for others who are faced with multiple sclerosis and its challenges, and their families. YOU CAN TRULY AFFECT THE COURSE OF THIS DISEASE AND THE COURSE OF YOUR LIFE.

Since grade school we have been told to get plenty of exercise and to eat properly. Much of what we were taught about eating properly was not correct. Don't accept what you are told without "remembering" the truth. Much of the information we are taught is fed to us by the pharmaceutical companies "and by our agricultural industry" which will be discussed at length at a later time. The Food and Drug Administration (FDA) and the United States Department of Agriculture (USDA) are very much controlled by the people they are intended to regulate. This is like "having the fox guard the hen house."

Today, walking and exercising is part of my everyday life. I am still learning new things about eating, almost every day it seems. Much that we have learned is beneficial.

I often didn't follow great advice that I had from teachers, parents and other adults. Sometimes I think about how my life would have been different if I had been taking care of my health since I was twenty. Of course, that same reasoning could apply to many areas of my life if I were doing it over. The truth is that I chose my own path. On the surface it certainly seems that I would have made different choices. Why do you choose a particular graduate school? Maybe it is because you want to learn certain things. Some things I obviously needed to learn. Much of this has been really difficult.

I was born into a family situation that insured lots of stress. I lived my life in a way that included stress for many years after that. Each took its toll on my mind and body. In the same way, poor eating habits and lack of attention to my health played a huge part in my health problems.

I feel blessed in many ways. I had the opportunity to learn a lot as I was struggling through all of this. I could have been taking all of the medicine that the pharmaceuticals throw at the problem. There is no way to tell what serious side effects may have accompanied those medicines.

I encourage you not to accept at face value, all we have been taught or all our doctors have been taught. There is lots to learn and it takes effort. Faith can play an incredible part in the healing process and in our lives. I feel compelled to remind you that our pharmaceutical companies are motivated by profits and not by finding a cure for multiple sclerosis.

They are the most profitable companies, by far, in our country. Profit is their motivation. Their stockholders invested to make a profit, not to be altruistic. I am glad that I did not take their medicine for my Multiple Sclerosis. I am glad that I realized that I could greatly affect the condition of my mind and body.

Most of my multiple sclerosis symptoms are gone or, are not very noticeable. I was fortunate not to have taken medicine that was offered. I was fortunate to have a neurologist who continued to see me when I declined to take medicine.

I was fortunate to find a church that assisted me with a great learning and healing experience and friends to assist me on my journey. One direct effect of this was my exposure to many great books that I have read. I have managed to give credit to some of these wonderful writers.

Being healed and feeling well is a worthwhile objective. Being happy with who you are and where you are is necessary if you are to achieve this objective.

Be thankful for every moment that you have here. While working diligently to achieve good health, remain in a state of gratitude.

I have often been referred to as an "eternal optimist." This has led me into some real challenges. It has also kept me going when confronted with seemingly, overwhelming odds.

Persistence and perseverance can go a long way toward reaching your goals. Don't' let the length and difficulty of the journey discourage you from taking the trip. Take small steps; have reachable goals.

When I started walking in the mall, I could see the goal line – that spot about 150 feet away with a bench were I could sit for a moment before going again.

The end result of years of hard work has been the disappearance of my multiple sclerosis symptoms, along with the disappearance of plaque, or scar tissue, from my brain. This was accomplished without taking medication that has the potential to cause more problems than it solves.

Prayer, faith, a healthy diet, and lots of exercise all combine to create miracles. I can attest to that. Start creating miracles in your own life today. That begins with a thought. Now, create your own road map and have a wonderful journey!

> *The greatest discovery of my generation is that human beings, by changing the inner attitudes of their minds, can change the outer aspects of their lives.*
> — *William James*

> *The body is a great healer. The magnificent perfect creation is capable of healing itself in many, many instances.*
> — *Dr. Wayne Dyer*

End Notes

These two writers do us a great service in spotlighting the abuses of our pharmaceutical industry.

ANGELL, MARCIA: *THE TRUTH ABOUT THE DRUG COMPANIES: HOW THEY DECEIVE US AND WHAT TO DO ABOUT IT*, Random House, 2004

HALEY, DANIEL: *POLITICS IN HEALING*, Potomac Valley Press, Washington, D.C., 2000

* - * - *

I give special thanks to these writers for helping to shape my own healing process (in alphabetical order):

FILLMORE, MYRTLE: *HOW TO LET GOD HELP YOU*, Unity Books, Unity Village, Missouri, 1956, Eleven printings through 1991.

JAFOLLA, MARY ALICE: *THE SIMPLE TRUTH, A BASIC GUIDE TO METAPHYSICS*, Unity Books, Unity Village, Missouri, 1982, by Unity School of Christianity.

PONDER, CATHERINE: *THE DYNAMIC LAWS OF HEALING*, DeForss & Company, Marina Del Rey, California, 1966

SIEGEL, BERNIE S., M.D.: *LOVE, MEDICINE & MIRACLES*, Harper & Row Publishers, New York, N.Y., 1986

WALSH, NEALE DONALD: *CONVERSATIONS WITH GOD*, G.P,. Puntam's Sons, New York, N.Y., 1996

WITHERSPOON, THOMAS E.: *MYRTLE FILLMORE, MOTHER OF UNITY*, Unity Book, Unity Village, Missouri, 1977

* ‑ * ‑ *

I used short quotes from three different writers who compiled books of them. From those three writers I could have had a quote on each page. Those compilations were by:

1) Dr. Wayne Dyer

2) Bernie S. Siegel, M.D.

3) Rosemarie Jarsk

Many of these quotes are from people in the medical community over a long period of time. I found it both sad, and interesting, that over the years, so much has been forgotten by so many. "First do no harm."

* - * - *

Recommended Reading

My healing process covered many years, more than a decade. I did lots of reading. Listed here are many of the books that were enlightening, educational, and strengthened my resolve to take charge of my own health. I recommend any, or all, of these books. I remind the reader, again, that MS played havoc with my body for years before it disappeared. I wish that I could have packed all of this knowledge into my book. All I could do was tell my story; these writers contributed greatly to my healing (in alphabetical order):

CHOPRA, DEEPAK, M.D.: _PERFECT HEALTH, THE COMPLETE MIND BODY GUIDE_, Three Rivers Press, NY, NY, 2000.

COHEN, ALAN: _DARE TO BE YOURSELF_, Alan Cohen Publications, and Random House, NY, NY, 1991.

COHEN, ALAN: _WHY YOUR LIFE SUCKS, AND WHAT YOU CAN DO ABOUT IT_, Jodere Group, 2002, and Cohen Publications, 2004, Bantam, 2005.

DOSSEY, LARRY, M.D.: _MEANING AND MEDICINE, A DOCTOR'S TALES OF BREAKTHROUGH AND HEALING_, Bantam, 1991.

DOSSEY, LARRY, M.D.: _HEALING WORDS: THE POWER OF PRAYER AND THE PRACTICE OF MEDICINE_, Harper, San Francisco, 1993.

Dr. Dossey has written several widely read books. These two greatly impacted my journey and my recovery.

DYER, WAYNE, PH.D.: _THE POWER OF INTENTION, LEARNING TO CO-CREATE YOUR WORLD YOUR WAY_, Hay House, 2004

DYER, WAYNE, PH.D.: <u>INSPIRATION, YOUR ULTIMATE CALLING</u>, Hay House, 2006

Dr. Dyer is truly the most prolific writer that I have ever encountered. I will not even attempt to list all that he has written. Hay House has been his publisher for years. Fortunately, I have read almost every book he has written. **These two were truly powerful.**

HAWKINS, DAVID R., M.D., PH.D.: <u>POWER VS. FORCE</u>, Hay House, Carlsbad, California, 1995, 2002.

HAY, LOUISE L.: <u>HEAL YOUR BODY</u>, Hay House, Inc., Carson, CA 1982

HAY, LOUISE L.: <u>YOU CAN HEAL YOUR LIFE</u>, Hay House, Inc., Carson, CA 1984

HAY, LOUISE L.: <u>THE POWER IS WITHIN YOU</u>, Hay House, Inc., Carson, CA 1991

MULLER, WAYNE: <u>HOW THEN SHALL WE LIVE?</u>, Bantam books, NY, NY, 1996

RUIZ, DON MIGUEL: <u>THE FOUR AGREEMENTS</u>, Amber Allen Publishing, Inc., San Rafael, California, 1997.

RYCE, DR. MICHAEL: _WHY IS THIS HAPPENING TO ME … AGAIN?! … AND WHAT YOU CAN DO ABOUT IT!_, Published by Dr. Michael Ryce, Theodosis, Missouri, 1997.

SHEALY, NORMAN C., PH.D. and **MYSS, CARDINE M., M.A.**: _THE CREATION OF HEALTH, THE EMOTIONAL, PSYCHOLOGICAL, AND SPIRITUAL RESPONSES THAT PROMOTE HEALTH AND HEALING_, Stillpoint Publishing, Walpole, NH, 1988.

TOLLE, EKHART: _A NEW EARTH: AWAKENING TO YOUR LIFE'S PURPOSE_, Penguin Group, 2006.